Quick Reference to Triage

Quick Reference to Triage

Valerie G. A. Grossman, BSN, CEN, CCRN

Clinical Leader
Emergency Department
F.F. Thompson Hospital
Canandaigua, New York

Community Pediatric Telephone Triage
University of Rochester
Rochester, New York

Lippincott

Philadelphia • New York • Baltimore

Acquisitions Editor: Susan M. Glover, RN, MSN
Coordinating Editorial Assistant: Bridget Blatteau
Project Editor: Tom Gibbons
Senior Production Manager: Helen Ewan
Production Coordinator: Pat McCloskey
Design Coordinator: Brett MacMaughton
Indexer: Victoria Boyle

Library of Congress Cataloging in Publications Data
Grossman, Valerie G. A.
   Quick reference to triage / Valerie G.A. Grossman.
      p.   cm.
   Includes bibliographical references and index.
   ISBN 0-7817-1861-9 (alk. paper)
   1. Triage (Medicine)—Handbooks, manuals, etc.   I. Title.
   [DNLM: 1. Triage handbooks.   2. Emergency Medical Services
handbooks.   3. Emergencies handbooks.   WX 39G878q 1999]
   RC86.8.G76 1999
   616.02′5—dc21
   DNLM/DLC
   for Library of Congress   98-385465
                                                           CIP

Care has been taken to confirm the accuracy of the information presented and to describe generally accepted practices. However, the authors, editors, and publisher are not responsible for errors or omissions or for any consequences from application of the information in this book and make no warranty, express or implied, with respect to the contents of the publication.

The authors, editors and publisher have exerted every effort to ensure that drug selection and dosage set forth in this text are in accordance with current recommendations and practice at the time of publication. However, in view of ongoing research, changes in government regulations, and the constant flow of information relating to drug therapy and drug reactions, the reader is urged to check the package insert for each drug for any change in indications and dosage and for added warnings and precautions. This is particularly important when the recommended agent is a new or infrequently employed drug.

Some drugs and medical devices presented in this publication have Food and Drug Administration (FDA) clearance for limited use in restricted research settings. It is the responsibility of the health care provider to ascertain the FDA status of each drug or device planned for use in their clinical practice.

9   8   7   6   5   4   3   2

REVIEWERS

Samuel S. Bean, MS, RN
Wayne Regional Orthopaedic Associates
Immediate Past Director of Emergency Nursing
Mycrs Community Hospital
Sodus, New York

Julie Briggs, RN, BSN, MHA
Administrative Director
Emergency Department
Good Samaritan Community Healthcare
Puyallup, Washington

Frank J. Edwards, MD, FACEP
Clinical Assistant Professor of Emergency Medicine
University of Rochester School of Medicine
Director, Division of Community and Rural Emergency Medicine of ViaHealth
Rochester, New York

Kevin Hanna, MD
Community and Rural Emergency Medicine
  of ViaHealth
Myers Community Hospital
Sadus, New York

R. Thomas Huntley
Public Health Regional Supervisor
Sexually Transmitted Disease Control Program
New York State Health Department
Syracuse, New York

Merrill Beth Kotok, RN C
Fetal Monitoring Unit
University of Rochester
Strong Memorial Hospital
Rochester, New York

Neal L. McGregor PhD(c)
Professor of Religion and Business
Graceland College
Lamoni, Iowa

Margaret M. McMahon, RN, MN, CEN
Clinical Educator
Emergency Services
Atlantic City Medical Center
Atlantic City, New Jersey

Susan Spinello, CRNP, MSN, CEN, CCRN
Clinical Specialist
Emergency Department
University of Pennsylvania Medical Center
Philadelphia, Pennsylvania

Joseph Stamm, OD, FAAO
Private Practice
Clinical Associate, Department of Ophthalmology
University of Rochester School of Medicine
Rochester, New York

Marcia Ullman, MS, RN
Associate Professor of Psychiatric Nursing
State University of New York
College at Brockport
Brockport, New York

ILLUSTRATOR

John F. Aarne
Freelance Artist
Homer, New York

PREFACE

Keeping pace with the ever-changing health care arena is a challenge for experienced health care professionals. The venture of entering a new environment in health care can seem overwhelming.

A common thread for anyone entering a patient care setting as the new team member is the need for user-friendly information. Facilities are well supplied with policy and procedure books and reference material for caregivers to refer to when clinical or administrative questions arise. New orientees and seasoned colleagues are often encouraged to create and carry "note cards" in their pockets. These note cards are highly individualized to the learning and practicing needs of each person.

Quick Reference to Triage, in essence, takes those note cards and compiles them into one source. It features a user-friendly format, allowing the busy health care professional to glance quickly at a page and determine immediately what should be assessed and considered for each patient. Over time, some of this material will be committed to memory...and some won't.

For consistency, the wording of the text refers to the emergency department setting. The material in this book is entirely appropriate for urgent care centers, private offices, schools, home health care agencies, prisons, and any other outpatient setting where patient assessment and triage occurs.

ACKNOWLEDGMENTS

The completion of this book is due to the commitment and dedication of many wonderful people.

First, I would like to share my sincere appreciation for my writing mentors; Cynthia Olmstead, Mary Salbrici, Donna Ojanen Thomas, Frank Edwards, Sam Bean, Peter Marchant, and Marcia Ullman. These incredible visionaries invested their time and expertise in me, inspiring me to develop into the writer I am today.

Secondly, I am most grateful to my panel of reviewers and the staff at Lippincott Williams & Wilkins. These groups of dedicated professionals maintained high standards and expectations for this text, were meticulously attentive to detail and deadlines, and believed in the investment this book required of all of us.

Lastly, a standing ovation for the life partners God has blessed me with: John and Marie Aarne (my folks)...my father for creating the artwork in this text and to my mother for standing with us all these years; my best friend and husband, Alan, who, no matter what mountain we are climbing, believes in me; and my daughters, Nicole and Sarah Lynn, who are my constant inspiration and delight...who look forward to each of my published works...and who plan to co-author my next book with me. You are all the greatest.

CONTENTS

PART III

PART IV

PART V

Triage Process

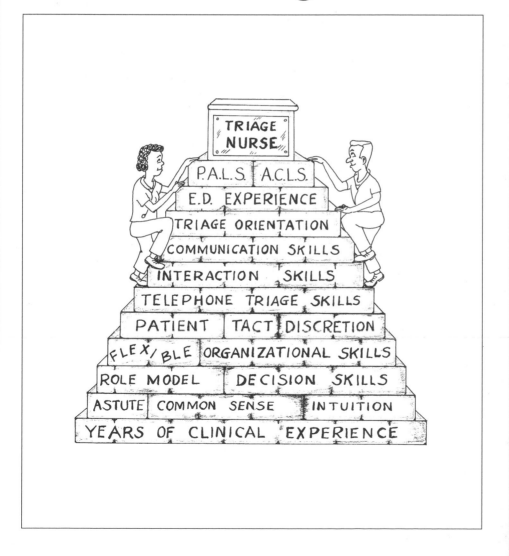

Notes

► FROM BATTLEFIELD TO FACILITY

Triage is derived from the French word, "trier," meaning to sort out. It was first used by the French military during World War I, when victims were sorted and classified according to the type and urgency of their conditions for the purpose of determining medical treatment priorities. The military intent was to provide care to the most treatable of casualties for a rapid return of soldiers to the war front. Combat triage was guided by the adage "the best for the most with the least by the fewest" (Simoneau, 1985). Critical patients requiring extensive resources received delayed medical care.

Lessons learned from wartime triaging are useful in the public sector. Triage is now used to organize the medical care available during disasters and mass casualty situations, and in emergency departments, urgent care centers, physicians' offices, and over the telephone.

Emergency Department (ED) use of triage systems began in the early 1960s, when the demand for emergency services outpaced available emergency resources. Emergency department space, equipment, and personnel were not adequate to handle the explosive increase in the number of emergency department visits.

The rise in the number of ED visits was the result of many factors, including:

Δ More patients seeking treatment for nonurgent conditions
Δ Patients with no other access to health care
Δ An increasing population sustaining a higher acuity of acute and chronic illnesses
Δ The negative impact from the rising use of illicit drugs
Δ An increase in the incidence of violent crime and trauma

As the use of emergency departments increased and the waiting times became longer, the triage process evolved as a way to effectively separate those patients requiring immediate medical attention from those who could wait. Triage in health care facilities differs in both purpose and function from that on the battlefield or at the disaster site. ED triage has become a major component of the emergency medical system and an expected standard of emergency nursing practice.

The primary goals of an effective ED triage system are to:

Δ *Quickly* identify those patients with emergent, life-threatening conditions
Δ Regulate the flow of patients through the Emergency Department (ED)
Δ Provide direction to visitors and other health care professionals

An efficient triage system increases the quality of patient care delivered, shortens the length of a patient's stay, and decreases patient waiting time by combining immediate assessment and interventions. Organized triage categories are used to rate patient acuity, and standards are followed for assessment, planning, and intervention. Protocols are used for the initiation of specific diagnostic tests, medication administration, and treatments.

The advantages of triage follow.

Δ The patient is greeted by a registered professional nurse, which establishes immediate communication, rapport, and sensitivity to the patient's and family's needs. The image of the facility is enhanced through positive client perceptions.
Δ Patient stress and anxiety are reduced when there is immediate contact with the nurse. The patient gains comfort knowing he or she is "in the system."

Δ Initial patient communication with the hospital, via the triage nurse, does not concern insurance or the ability to pay. This instills confidence in the patient that the ED is genuinely concerned with health problems and less concerned with ability to pay for the service received.

Δ Treatment of the patient requiring immediate care is expedited by the use of an acuity category system.

Δ Immediate assessment and documentation of patient problems are provided while certain diagnostic procedures and treatments can be initiated without delay.

Δ Continuous reassessment of the ED patient who is waiting to be seen, and continued communication with waiting family and friends, ensure the delivery of quality care.

QUALITIES OF THE TRIAGE NURSE

The triage nurse is the first health care professional seen by the patient in the ED. Hospital surveys have shown that patient satisfaction with the emergency department and the hospital as a whole can be influenced by the initial encounter with the triage nurse (McMillan, 1986).

The triage nurse must be sensitive to the patient's perception of the *health crisis* that brought him or her to the ED. The triage nurse must help the patient regain control and increase the understanding of his or her own health care role. Triage begins the process of managing a person's crisis instead of merely reacting to the situation.

Essential to the building of rapport between the triage nurse and the patient is the patient's first impression. The triage nurse has one opportunity to make a first impression on the patient. While in the waiting room or approaching the registration desk, the patient has the opportunity to view the triage nurse "on stage." The patient begins to develop an impression of the nurse before the first interaction even occurs. For this reason, it is vital for the triage nurse to act in a professional manner 100% of the time. The patient needs to know that the nurse is a genuinely concerned expert who is ready to assist in the patient's health care.

When greeting an incoming patient, the triage nurse must introduce her- or himself to the patient. Most patients will be unaware of what a triage nurse is or what the process for being cared for in the ED will be. This is an excellent opportunity for the triage nurse to "open the hospitality door" for the patient, begin the triage assessment, and educate the patient as to what can be expected during the ED visit.

The triage nurse acts as a positive influence for the patient by offering comfort and by communicating with the person in crisis. A guiding hand, gentle voice tone, warm smile, and attention to basic comfort needs (i.e., offering to carry coats or a parent's diaper bag) create an environment of true caring for the patient and family members.

Multisituational organization and communication skills are essential for the triage nurse. Although the nurse may have to handle many different chaotic events at once, he or she must always make the patient in the triage room feel important. The triage nurse must be skilled in quality customer service, able to balance it all with graceful expertise—ringing telephones, ambulances, police, hospital colleagues, news media, and those in the waiting room.

The triage nurse encounters many persons in the course of a shift. An unbiased and open mind is essential. The nurse must practice in an accepting manner, regardless of the cultural, religious, or social differences of the patients seeking care in the ED.

Much of the background for triage nursing is drawn from common sense. The basis for this comes from years of clinical experience, a broad range of nursing and medical knowledge, and extensive experience in dealing with emergency patients. These experiences, coupled with a working knowledge of ED routines, policies, and procedures, lead to a competent and efficient triage nurse.

The general qualifications strongly recommended for all ED nurses, and especially those performing in the triage role, include:

Δ 6 months of emergency nursing experience
Δ Demonstrated mastery of the hospital ED's competency-based orientation program
Δ Advanced Cardiac Life Support certification
Δ Pediatric Advanced Life Support certification
Δ Emergency Nurses Pediatric Course completion
Δ Trauma Nurse Core Curriculum
Δ Precision assessment skills
Δ Certification in Emergency Nursing
Δ Working knowledge of intradepartmental policies
Δ Ability to supervise others and delegate appropriately
Δ Understanding of local emergency services (ambulance, police, helicopter, etc.)
Δ Excellent telephone triage skills

Personal qualifications include:

Δ Ability to utilize interpersonal and communication skills
Δ Ability to work collaboratively and interact well with others
Δ Flexibility and adaptability, to meet the challenge of rapidly changing situations
Δ Ability to act as a role model
Δ Ability to utilize decision-making skills
Δ Ability to anticipate future events and plan for potential occurrences
Δ Mature understanding of conflict resolution
Δ Well-developed skills in handling patients with communication barriers such as:
  • Non–English speaking
  • Expressive aphasia
  • Intoxication from alcohol or other drugs
  • Belligerent, hostile, or aggressive behavior
  • Hearing or sight impairment
  • Mental handicap
  • Hysterical, crying, or panicky emotional state

To be a good triage nurse is to be a skilled, astute, compassionate health care professional with a great deal of common sense and intuition. It is one of the ultimate challenges in emergency nursing.

TRIAGE "HOW TO'S"

The triage evaluation is an assessment process that collects objective and subjective information. The interview and physical assessment at triage must be reasonably comprehensive yet fit into a 2- to 5-minute time period. A complete head-to-toe assessment is usually neither feasible nor necessary.

The triage nurse practices within guidelines established by hospital, state, and federal agencies. In order to maintain compliance with established laws and regulations, the ED nurse performing triage is held to a degree of excellence that must always be maintained.

All patients presenting for care should be triaged on arrival (usually within 5 minutes) and receive a triage evaluation by the nurse prior to speaking with registration personnel. Patients presenting to the ED are always entitled to receive care in the ED, regardless of ability to pay for service.

During times of extremely high patient volume, when the existing triage system is overloaded and patients are waiting an excessive amount of time to be evaluated by the nurse, the triage nurse on duty is responsible for gaining assistance in the triage area. Each facility should have an overflow procedure in place that may include:

△ Having the ED technician obtain vital signs for each patient in triage while the nurse continues patient assessments
△ Requesting assistance from another ED nurse on duty
△ Requesting assistance from the ED charge nurse or other supervisory person

The triage assessment is the first segment of care the patient receives. It provides enough data to determine patient acuity and any immediate physiological, psychological, psychosocial, or educational needs. Additionally, the information gathered by the triage nurse can be used for starting treatment or diagnostic testing from the triage office following established protocols that the facility may have in place. These may include x-rays, administration of antipyretics, or diphtherial tetanus immunization.

The triage nurse is responsible for assigning patients to an appropriate treatment area. In cases in which there is a question as to the level of triage acuity, the choice should be made toward the more urgent assignment of care.

The triage nurse or the ED nurse taking over the care of that patient should ensure that reassessment occurs for each patient waiting to be seen by the physician. The assigned acuity level must be updated continually to include a change in the patient status or new information provided by the patient or family.

► HOSPITAL RECEPTIONIST

In many hospitals, the first employee a client meets is the receptionist at the front desk, usually situated at or close to the front entrance. This person is generally responsible for greeting the incoming patient or visitor in a friendly manner, welcoming the patient to the facility, and assisting him or her with directions.

When the person presenting to this desk is sick or injured and seeking directions to the emergency department, the hospital receptionist must carefully guide the way. There are times, however, when the patient should not continue toward the emergency department without the assistance of a trained medical person in attendance.

The hospital receptionist is generally untrained in the recognition of medical emergencies. Training and on-the-job experience increase the receptionist's ability to determine those patients who "look sicker" than most.

The following Table is designed to assist the hospital receptionist in determining how the patient should be guided to the ED or if a medically trained person should be contacted immediately. It is based on the complaint (usually in one or two words) that the patient describes to the receptionist on arrival.

Guidelines for the Recognition of Medical Emergencies

Call for Emergency Response "Code Blue"	Call RN Immediately	Send Patient to Triage Area Notify RN
Lifeless child carried in	Chest pain	Nausea, vomiting, diarrhea
Lifeless adult carried in	Difficulty breathing	"Cold" symptoms
	Gunshot wound	Minor wound, cut, bite
	Stab wound	Sore throat
	Seizure	Earache
	Massive bleeding	Bruise
	Difficulty staying awake	Minor sprain, strain
	Severe allergic reaction	
	Attempted suicide	
	Active labor/childbirth	
	Exposed broken bone	
	Violent patient	
	Eye injury (vision loss)	
	Large burn	
	Fever over 104°F	
	MVA/multiple trauma victim	

Points to remember:

- Call the RN if there is any question.
- Help the patient who needs assistance (wheelchair, etc.).
- Receptionists must not triage the patient or render medical advice.

INTERVIEW

The triage nurse should always begin the triage interview by introducing her- or himself by name and title. This provides the patient with the following.

△ Confidence that he or she is receiving care from a registered professional nurse
△ The opportunity of open communication with the RN
△ An additional degree of comfort, knowing he or she can now identify with a member of the team by name

The triage interview is the basis for gathering data and making clinical decisions regarding the patient's acuity and need for intervention. The nurse elicits:

△ Chief complaints
△ Subjective and objective information pertinent to the presenting problem by utilizing the sense of:
  - sight
  - smell
  - listening

- intuition
- touch

LOOK at the patient.

Δ Keen observation reveals:
- fear
- anxiety
- deformities
- respiratory problems
- obvious bleeding
- abnormal gait
- poor personal hygiene
- changes in skin color
- innumerable other signs

SMELL the patient's odors.

Δ The seasoned triage nurse is able to identify:
- alcohol
- marijuana
- ketone bodies
- incontinence
- ingested substances or poisons
- purulent infectious process

Δ The nurse must be sensitive to a host of smells that indicate different directions of treatment modalities.

LISTEN to what the patient and family are saying and to what they *are not* saying.

Δ The triage nurse uses the sense of hearing to assess:
- pain
- fear
- gross rales
- coughing
- shortness of breath
- a muffled voice
- family dynamics
- other indicators of a problem

TOUCH is instrumental in many ways.

Δ The sense of touch can assess:
- temperature
- sensation
- moisture
- "where it hurts"
- capillary refill
- soft tissue swelling

Δ By taking a radial pulse, the nurse can assess heart rate, possible cardiac arrhythmia, skin temperature, turgor, and so on.

Δ Touch can also be:

- psychologically therapeutic
- used as an evaluation tool
- used to communicate

Intuition plays a strong role in decisions made during triage.

Δ Intuition is a "sixth sense" that a patient:

- is experiencing a problem that is more serious than it appears
- is at risk for certain complications
- needs particular attention to a set of symptoms

Δ This *unexplained sense* that results with the nurse entering the patient into the ED as a more acute patient is based on:

- in-depth knowledge of diseases and injuries
- educational opportunities encountered throughout one's career
- years of experience
- CQI of presentations during triage evaluation of patients
- a wide range of patients, disease processes, injuries, and variable presentation seen over a period of many years (Handysides, 1996)

The triage interview should always be conducted with open-ended questions and an open mind in order to gather pertinent information.

PHYSICAL ASSESSMENT

Physical assessment accompanies the triage interview and often occurs while the nurse is obtaining the history. The physical assessment should be rapid, concise, and focused.

The nurse performing triage should always begin with the primary survey (airway, breathing, and circulation), followed by the secondary survey. The use of the PQRSTT mnemonic is helpful in systematically evaluating the presenting system:

P = Provoking factors   What makes it (pain, breathing, etc.) worse?
What makes it better?
Any known trauma or injury?

Q = Quality of pain   What does it feel like?
Does the patient use descriptive words, such as burning, stabbing, crushing, or tearing?

R = Region/Radiation

Where is the pain?
Is it in one spot?
Does it start in one spot and travel to another?
Ask the patient to point to where it hurts using one finger.

S = Severity of pain

If the patient were to describe the pain with a number from 1 to 10, with 1 being the least severe and 10 being the worst pain imaginable, what number would the patient give this pain?

T = Time

When did this start?
How long have the symptoms persisted?
How long did it last?
Has it ever happened before?

T = Treatment

Has the patient taken any medication to treat this?
What time was the last dose?
Has the patient done anything to treat him- or herself?
What has or has not worked for the patient?

By using the eyes, ears, nose, hands, and intuition, the triage nurse is able to have an accurate idea whether this patient requires immediate care or can wait the turn in line. Remember, make a triage decision, not a diagnosis.

BASIC TRIAGE ASSESSMENT

All patients presenting to the ED have a routine triage assessment performed, including a primary and a focused secondary assessment.

All findings must be accurately documented.

Depending on facility policy, obtain the following information:

Δ Patient name (ask patient for correct spelling)

Δ Date and time of initial patient contact with triage nurse

Δ Mode of arrival (walk, wheelchair, car, or ambulance)

Δ Age in years (if >2 years old) or in months (if <24 months)

Δ Chief complaint of the patient, usually two to three quoted words from patient

Δ Brief triage history and physical assessment per protocol

Δ Current medication taken by patient, including over-the-counter medication, prescription medication, tobacco use, alcohol use, and illicit drug use

Δ Allergies to medication, including the reaction (rash, respiratory distress, etc.)

- Some facilities use red ink for documenting allergies
- Assess for latex allergy on all patients by asking, "Have you ever developed itching, burning, swelling, or hives after blowing up a balloon or wearing rubber gloves?"

Δ Immunization status for all patients < 18 years old per protocol and last dT for all patients >18 years old regardless of complaint

Δ The first day of the last normal menstrual period (LNMP) for all women of childbearing age

Δ Weight for all pediatric patients

Δ Vital signs, per departmental policy

Δ Triage acuity assessment and documentation per protocol

Δ Glasgow Coma Scale (GCS) and/or Trauma Score (TS) for all trauma patients, altered LOC, head injury patients, and so on

Δ Signature of triage nurse (including first initial, last name, and credentials)

ORTHOSTATIC VITAL SIGNS

Orthostatic vital signs can be a beneficial assessment tool for the triage nurse in assigning acuity levels to triaged patients. Orthostatic vital signs should be assessed on all patients who present with:

Δ Vomiting
Δ Fever
Δ Diarrhea
Δ Abdominal pain
Δ Dizziness
Δ Syncope
Δ Weakness
Δ Bleeding (vaginal)

Caution: If a patient looks hemodynamically unstable, has a possible or probable spinal injury, or has an altered level of consciousness, the triage nurse should defer obtaining orthostatic vital signs until *after* the patient is evaluated by the physician.

To perform this procedure:

1. The patient should rest in the supine position for 3–5 minutes.
2. After this rest, obtain blood pressure (BP) and pulse with the patient in the supine position.
3. Slowly assist the patient to a sitting position, with feet dangling over the bed side.
4. Allow the patient to remain in this sitting position for 1 minute.
5. After this rest, obtain a BP and pulse with the patient in the sitting position.
6. Slowly assist the patient to a standing position.
7. Allow the patient to remain in the standing position for 1 minute.
8. After this rest, obtain a BP and pulse.
9. Assess how the patient tolerated the procedure (asymptomatic, became dizzy, etc.).

To document this procedure:

1. Indicate the time of the procedure.
2. Indicate if the patient experienced symptoms during the procedure.
3. Document each BP and pulse for each position.

Example:

8:30 AM	lying:	140/68	HR 82
	sitting	136/66	HR 90
	standing	128/62	HR 100

Stick figures, instead of the written word, may be used for documentation purposes when describing the different positions.

A "positive" result would show:

Δ a fall in the systolic blood pressure of >20 mmHg
Δ a fall in the diastolic blood pressure of >10 mmHg
Δ a rise in the pulse of >20 beats per minute

Orthostatic vital signs can be partially utilized in the triage room, especially during times of high volume and acuity in the department. By performing the sitting and standing portion of this procedure, the triage nurse is able to assess the patient's acuity level more precisely and make a more accurate decision regarding the priority of care.

Orthostatic vital signs are also utilized during the ongoing care of patients. The nurse may decide to utilize them as a part of the ongoing assessment process of the patient in addition to their use during triage or when specifically requested by the physician.

Orthostatic vital signs should be considered as part of the reassessment of:

Δ Patients receiving IV hydration

Δ Patients who had "positive" orthostatic vital signs on arrival

Δ Patients who received medication that could cause drowsiness or other central nervous system (CNS) depression

▶ DOCUMENTATION

The triage process is complete when the information elicited during the assessment process has been fully and accurately documented. Documentation on the patient's ED chart is crucial to support the decisions and actions of the triage nurse and the ED staff.

All pertinent information gathered during the triage process (interview history and physical assessment) must be documented. Pertinent negatives may also be listed, such as "denies nausea, vomiting, or fever." These are important pieces of necessary information when focusing on the patient's condition.

If nursing interventions took place during triage, documentation should reflect those. It is essential that every nursing intervention from the administration of antipyretics to the seclusion of a patient in a quiet room be appropriately recorded on the patient's medical record.

▶ ASSIGNING ACUITY

Δ Triage acuity categories represent:
  - the acuity of each patient's condition
  - the anticipated amount of nursing care the patient will need while in the ED
  - a continuum in which one patient presents more emergent than another

Δ In cases where there is a question as to the level of triage acuity, the choice should be made toward the *more serious* category of care.
  - Each Emergency Department should have its own patient classification system in place, which can be located in the ED policy book.
  - Determining the acuity category for those patients in the middle of the continuum is a challenge for the triage nurse.

Δ The triage nurse should carefully consider those age-fragile patients (<12 months or >60 years old) who may be less able to tolerate the more simple injuries and illnesses, and may adjust the patient's acuity level to a more serious category.

Δ If a patient presents with more than one chief complaint, the triage nurse must individually address each of the patient's concerns.

- The nurse may opt to place this patient in a higher acuity category, as the client's ED medical evaluation will probably be more detailed.

Δ The triage nurse applies subjective and objective data gathered to determine triage categories. For instance:

- On the basis of practical knowledge gained through experience and training, certain signs and symptoms trigger the triage nurse's suspicion toward a particular clinical impression. For example, the 64-year-old male with chest pain and shortness of breath is classified as emergent because the nurse knows the probability of myocardial infarction in this patient and its potential complications.
- Discovery of a sign or symptom that will result in a poor outcome unless immediate care is rendered warrants a particular acuity category. For example, profuse bleeding or the presence of stridor directs the nurse to triage the patient as emergent.
- A standardized approach that promotes consistency and reliability throughout the ED nursing staff is attained by the triage nurse following established guidelines and triage protocols to determine the accurate triage acuity category. These guidelines promote early initiation of simple diagnostics, treatments, and patient teaching.

Δ It cannot be stressed enough that acuity categories are only a guideline.

- If the triage nurse believes that a patient needs to be placed at a higher level of acuity, it is within the realm of responsibilities of the triage nurse to do so.

Δ The triage nurse also must be careful of those patients who repeatedly visit the ED with minor complaints.

- Most psychoneurotic patients ultimately die from organic disease.
- We remember the story about the boy who cried wolf. We are now in a position to adapt and care for these patients who may not always be the easiest or most pleasant individuals.

Δ Patients who return to the ED within 72 hours are known to be high-risk patients.

- These patients may have a more progressive or severe medical condition than originally identified during their first visit.
- They may be dissatisfied with previous care received or seeking a second opinion.
- These patients must receive a complete medical screening exam by the ED physician *each* and *every* time they present to the ED.

Δ There are a variety of different triage models to follow using three, four, or five acuity categories.

Five-Level Acuity System

Level	Acuity	Treatment and Reassessment Time	Sample Conditions	
Level 1	Critical condition	Immediately	Cardiac arrest	Severe respiratory distress
			Seizure	Cardiac chest pain
			Anaphylaxis	Uncontrolled hemorrhage
			Coma	Severe head trauma
			Multiple trauma	Open chest/abdominal wound
			Profound shock	Poisoning with neurological changes
Level 2	Unstable condition	5–15 minutes	Major fracture	Overdose rapidly acting drug
			Severe headache	Tricyclic antidepressant
			Aggressive patient	Attempted suicide
			Major burn	Sexual assault survivor
			Acute asthma attack	Eye injury with loss of vision
			Active labor patient	Pregnant with active bleeding
Level 3	Potentially unstable	30–60 minutes	Alcohol intoxication	Abdominal pain
			Drug ingestion	Noncardiac chest pain
			Urinary retention	Severe emotional distress
			Renal calculi	Minor chest pain
			Laceration	Eye injury—vision intact
			Closed fracture	Bleeding, stable vital signs
Level 4	Stable condition	1–2 hours	Cystitis	Minor bites (human, insect, animal)
			Male STD	Vaginal discharge
			Sore throat	Constipation
			Abscess	Strain and sprain
			Minor burn	Earache
Level 5	Routine	4 hours	Routine physical	Suture removal, no complications
			Bruise	Prescription refill

Four-Level Acuity System

Level	Acuity	Treatment and Reassessment Time	Sample Conditions	
Level 1	Emergent	Immediately	Cardiac arrest	Severe respiratory distress
			Seizure	Cardiac chest pain
			Anaphylaxis	Uncontrolled hemorrhage
			Coma	Severe head trauma
			Multiple trauma	Open chest/abdominal wound
			Profound shock	Poisoning with neurological changes
			Major burns	Overdose rapidly acting drug
			Active labor patient	Tricyclic antidepressant
Level 2	Urgent	15–30 minutes	Major fracture	Sexual assault survivor
			Severe headache	Eye injury with loss of vision
			Aggressive patient	Severe abdominal pain
Level 3	Semiurgent	30–60 minutes	Alcohol intoxication	Abdominal pain
			Drug ingestion	Noncardiac chest pain
			Urinary retention	Severe emotional distress
			Renal calculi	Minor chest pain
			Laceration	Eye injury—vision intact
			Closed fracture	Bleeding, stable vital signs
Level 4	Nonurgent	1–2 hours	Cystitis	Minor bite (human, insect, animal)
			Male STD	Vaginal discharge
			Sore throat	Constipation
			Abscess	Strains and sprains
			Minor burn	Earache

Three-Level Acuity System

Level	Acuity	Treatment and Reassessment Time	Sample Conditions	
Level 1	Emergent	Immediately	Cardiac arrest	Severe respiratory distress
			Seizure	Cardiac chest pain
			Anaphylaxis	Uncontrolled hemorrhage
			Coma	Severe head trauma
			Multiple trauma	Open chest/abdominal wound
			Profound shock	Poisoning with neurological changes
			Major burn	Overdose rapidly acting drug
			Active labor patient	Tricyclic antidepressant
Level 2	Urgent	15–120 minutes	Alcohol intoxication	Abdominal pain
			Drug ingestion	Noncardiac chest pain
			Urinary retention	Severe emotional distress
			Renal calculi	Minor chest pain
			Laceration	Eye injury—vision intact
			Closed fracture	Bleeding, stable vital signs
Level 3	Nonurgent	2–4 hours	Rash	Strain and sprain
			Sore throat	Earache

PART II

Triage Guidelines

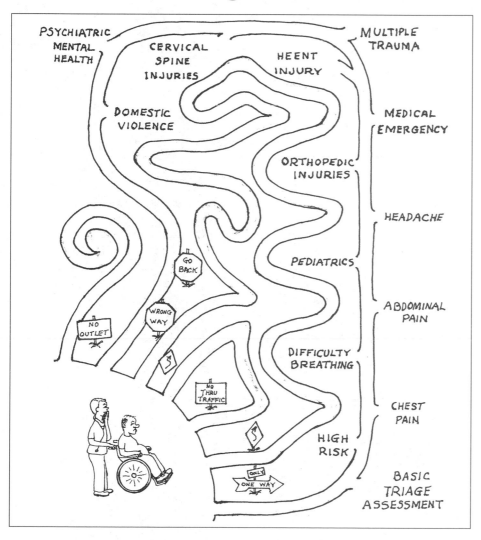

Notes

ABDOMINAL PAIN

Assessment

A. Obtain and record triage assessment that includes:
   1. Description of pain:
      △ **P**rovoking factors (what makes it better or worse?)
      △ **Q**uality of pain
      △ **R**egion/radiation
      △ **S**everity of pain (1–10 scale)
      △ **T**ime (onset, duration)
      △ **T**reatment (what has the patient already tried?)
   2. Associated symptoms:
      △ fever
      △ nausea
      △ vomiting
      △ diarrhea
      △ LNMP
      △ chest pain
      △ difficulty breathing
      △ last bowel movement
      △ urinary symptoms
      △ penile discharge
      △ gravid history
      △ vaginal discharge
   3. Past medical/surgical history:
      △ diabetes
      △ similar history of abdominal pain
      △ hypertension
      △ abdominal surgeries
      △ coronary artery disease
B. Complete basic triage assessment per protocol, and **document** accurately.
C. Obtain orthostatic vital signs as indicated.
D. Consider obtaining clean catch urine sample from female patients.
      △ if suspicion of urinary tract infection, a portion of the sample may be dipstick tested, with results recorded on triage note
      △ male patients presenting with possible STD symptoms **should not** obtain urine sample prior to physician exam

Immediate Care If

△ Age >50 years and/or any of the following:
- syncope (actual or near)
- hypertension

- arteriosclerotic heart disease
- diabetes
- aneurysm
- pain radiating into back or legs
- lightheadedness
- weakness/parathesias of legs
- systolic BP <100 or >160
- pulse >100 or <60
- any suspicion of AAA

Δ Heavy vaginal bleeding
Δ Blood in vomitus or stool (or suspicion of blood)
Δ Severe abdominal pain
Δ Unstable vital signs
Δ Persistent vomiting or profuse diarrhea:
- >18 hours in patients older than 6 years
- >12 hours in children less than 6 years old
- >8 hours since last void

Δ Referral by PMD with possible:
- acute abdomen
- intestinal obstruction

Differential Presentations of Abdominal Pain

Possible Diagnosis	Signs and Symptoms
Abdominal aortic aneurysm	• Asymptomatic until leakage or rupture occur • Abrupt onset of severe back, flank, or abdominal pain • Pulsatile abdominal mass, mottling of lower extremities, signs of shock
Appendicitis	• Diffuse pain in epigastric or periumbilical area for 1–2 days • Localization of pain over the right lower quadrant between the umbilicus and right iliac crest • Anorexia, nausea, vomiting, fever, tachycardia, pallor, peritoneal signs
Bowel obstruction	• Severe, cramp, colicky abdominal pain • Vomiting, constipation, hypotension, tachycardia, abdominal distention, hyperactive bowel sounds, fever
Cholecystitis (inflammation of gallbladder)	• Colicky discomfort in the right upper quadrant midepigastric area • Pain radiation to the shoulders and back • Nausea, vomiting, fever, tachycardia, tachypnea, abdominal guarding, jaundice, malaise
Cholelithiasis (presence of gallbladder stones)	• Severe, steady or colicky pain in the upper abdominal quadrant, often right-sided • Pain usually begins 3–6 hours after a large meal • Pain radiation to scapula, back, or right shoulder • Nausea, vomiting, dyspepsia, mild to moderate jaundice

Differential Presentations of Abdominal Pain (Continued)

Possible Diagnosis	Signs and Symptoms
Constipation/ fecal impaction	• Clinically defined as defecation less than three times per week • Each patient may interpret the symptoms differently • Fatigue, abdominal discomfort, headache, low back pain, anorexia, restlessness
Intussusception	• Paroxysms of acute Abdominal pain intermittent with episodes of being pain free • Currant jelly; mucus-type stools or rectal bleeding • Fever, lethargy, vomiting (food, mucus, fecal matter), dehydration
Pancreatitis	• Severe, constant upper quadrant midepigastric pain which radiates to the midback • Pain worsens when lying flat on back, relieved when lying on side with knees drawn up • Nausea, vomiting, fever, pallor, hypotension, tachycardia, tachypnea, restlessness, malaise, fatty or foul-smelling stools, abdominal distention, pulmonary crackles
Peritonitis	• Severe pain that gradually increases in intensity and worsens with movement • Riding in car, climbing stairs, or jumping on one foot greatly worsens pain • Radiation of pain to shoulder, back, or chest • Nausea, vomiting, fever, abdominal distention, rigidity, and tenderness
Renal calculi	• Location of stone depicts associated pain: flank, lower abdominal quadrant, low back, groin, testicular, labial, or urethral meatus • Pain radiation varies on stone location • Nausea, vomiting, pale, diaphoretic, marked restlessness, dehydration
Ruptured ovarian cyst	• Sudden severe, unilateral lower quadrant abdominal pain associated exercise or intercourse • Delayed or prolonged menstruation, vomiting, ascites, signs of peritonitis
Tubal pregnancy	• Intermittent diffuse abdominal pain • Radiation of pain to shoulder • Vaginal spotting/bleeding, syncope, dizziness, signs of peritonitis or shock
Urinary tract infection *Cystitis* *Pyelonephritis* *Prostatitis*	• Lower quadrant abdominal or pelvic pain • Dysuria, urinary frequency and urgency, fever, hematuria • Flank or back pain • Urinary frequency, dysuria, fever, malaise, nausea, vomiting, chills • Perineal aching, low back pain • Urinary frequency, dysuria, fever, malaise, urethral discharge, prostatic swelling
Ulcer (gastric, duodenal, esophageal)	• Colicky, burning, squeezing, pain in the epigastric or midback area • Pain intensity is variable, often begins 1–3 hours after meals, worsens at night • Nausea, vomiting, hematemesis, abdominal guarding, decreased or absent bowel sounds

ANKLE INJURIES

 Assessment

A. Obtain and record triage assessment that includes:
   1. What happened?
      Δ description of injury
      Δ mechanism of injury
         • inversion (foot bends inward, ankle falls outward)
         • eversion (foot bends outward, ankle bends inward)
   2. When did the injury occur?
   3. Can the patient put weight on the foot? ambulate?
   4. Where is the point of maximum tenderness?
   5. How is the circulation? (Check capillary refill and pedal pulses.)
B. Perform physical assessment of foot and ankle, by palpating:
      Δ lateral aspect of foot and ankle
      Δ medial aspect of foot and ankle
      Δ mid-foot region
      Δ fifth metatarsal
C. Complete remainder of basic triage assessment, and **document** completely.

 Immediate Care If

Δ marked deformity of the foot or ankle
Δ unstable foot or ankle joint
Δ absence of pulses or prolonged capillary refill
Δ open fracture

 Interventions

1. If triage assessment reveals a stable ankle, place patient in wheelchair, elevate affected leg, and apply ice to area.
   Δ Order x-ray of ankle (if your facility's protocol permits) if there is:
      • marked malleolar or submalleolar swelling/ecchymosis
      • history of severe pain when trying to bear weight
   Δ Order x-ray of foot (if your facility's protocol permits) if there is:
      • a crush type injury with mid-foot swelling
      • swelling over the base of the fifth metatarsal
   Δ Refrain from ordering x-ray if:
      • patient can reasonably bear weight
      • malleoli are not tender
      • no instability is noted

2. If triage assessment reveals an unstable ankle:
   Δ Place patient on a stretcher immediately
   Δ Apply ice to the area
   Δ Splint the joint with pillow or other available splint
   Δ Notify ED physician

► BURN TRAUMA

Facts

Δ Over 2 million burn injuries happen each year in the United States.
Δ Approximately 500,000 ED visits each year are from burn trauma.
Δ Of the 100,000 patients with major burns annually, approximately 6000 die as a result of their burn injury (American Burn Association, 1990).
Δ Different types of burn injury include:
- inhalation
- thermal
- electrical
- chemical
- radiation

Δ Burns initiate an inflammatory response of the affected area of the body, resulting in heat, redness, swelling, and pain.
Δ When the skin is burned, the following functions are altered:
- sensation
- skin regeneration
- body temperature
- conservation and balances of body fluids
- body image and self-esteem
- protection against infection and injury

General Issues

Assessment

A. Complete appropriate triage assessment protocol and **document** carefully.
  Δ basic triage assessment (important to determine underlying medical conditions)
  Δ multiple trauma (one-third of burn patients have other injuries)
  Δ pediatric trauma
  Δ domestic violence and child abuse
B. Assess burn wound.
  Δ type
  Δ location
  Δ blisters
  Δ appearance (e.g., blanching)
  Δ extent (rule of Nines—refer to diagram on p. 25)
  Δ depth (first-, second-, or third-degree—refer to table on p. 25)
C. Determine severity of burn injury and percentage of each type.

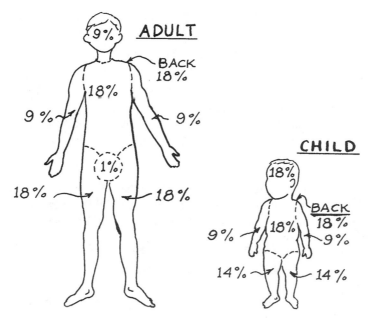

ADULT

9%

BACK 18%

18%

9%   9%

1%

18%   18%

CHILD

18%

BACK 18%

9%   18%   9%

14%   14%

Rule of Nines

Burn Identification

Depth	Degree	Appearance	Associated Pain	Healing Process
Partial thickness— epidermal	1st	Red and dry No blisters Blanches to pressure	Painful	3–5 days
Partial thickness— superficial	1st–2nd	Red to pale ivory color Weeping blisters Blanches to pressure	Increased sensitivity to: • Pain • Pressure • Temperature	10 days to 3 weeks
Partial thickness— deep	2nd–3rd	Mottled, white waxy Blisters Bullae	Depending on the depth, may be *very* painful or decreased sensitivity to: • Pain • Pressure • Temperature	Several weeks to months
Full thickness	3rd	Dry, white Charred, leathery Does not blanch	Absent sensitivity to: • Pain • Pressure • Temperature	Skin grafting required

Interventions

(vary depending on the severity and type of the burn injury)

1. Establish and maintain ABCs.
2. Insert intravenous access using large-bore catheters (14–16 ga) on unburned areas.
   Δ burned areas may be used if necessary, or may need cut down by MD.
3. Replace fluid volume deficit with lactated Ringer's solution (adult and child)
   Δ usual replacement formula for first 24 hours post–burn injury is *4cc LR × Kg × % of burn (up to 50% max)*
   Δ infuse as follows:
   - *First 8 hours* after burn: administer 1/2 of calculated IV replacement
   - *Second 8 hours* after burn: administer 1/4 of calculated IV replacement
   - *Third 8 hours* after burn: administer 1/4 of calculated IV replacement
4. Monitor and maintain urine output:
   Δ adults: 30–50 ml/hr (0.5–1.0 ml/Kg/hr)
   Δ children: <30 Kg: 1.0 ml/Kg/hr
5. Perform initial wound care:
   Δ if wound is still warm, apply cool, moist, sterile compress for no longer than 15 minutes to minor burns (<10% in age fragile, <15% in adults)
   Δ *never* place ice on a burn wound
   Δ consider pain management for all wound care procedures
   Δ cleanse minor burn wounds with a nondetergent soap; major burns will usually be cleansed by the receiving burn team
6. Consider use of documentation forms:
   Δ Pediatric Injury Assessment
   Δ Elder Abuse
   Δ Rules of Nines
7. Consider and arrange for the transfer of patient to a burn center using the criteria shown below.

Burn Center Transfer Criteria		
Age	*Depth*	*Total Body Surface Area (%)*
<10 years old	2nd and 3rd degree	>10
10–50 years old	2nd and 3rd degree	>20
>50 years old	2nd and 3rd degree	>10
Any age	3rd degree	>5

Inhalation Burn Injury

Assessment

1. Assess the patient for:
   Δ laryngeal spasm

Δ hoarseness
Δ singed facial hair
Δ dysphagia
Δ dyspnea
Δ cough
Δ ashen skin
Δ gray or black sputum
Δ carbonaceous sputum
Δ blisters in nose or mouth
Δ singed nasal hair
Δ uvual edema
Δ hypoxia
Δ pallor
Δ cyanosis
Δ soot in oropharynx

Carbon Monoxide Poisoning (Enclosed Exposure to Incomplete Combustion)

 Assessment

1. Determine what the patient was exposed to:
   Δ gas or propane
   Δ faulty furnace
   Δ fire
   Δ automobile exhaust
   Δ charcoal burner
   Δ stove
2. Obtain and evaluate carboxyhemoglobin saturation level (if needed)

Carboxyhemoglobin Saturation Levels	
Level (%)	Associated Indicators and Symptoms
0–5	Normal for nonsmokers
5–10	Normal for smokers
10–20	Headache, visual acuity impairment, irritability
20–30	Flushing, confusion
30–40	Nausea/vomiting, lack of coordination, dizziness, lethargy, ST segment depression
40–50	Chest pain, tachycardia, tachypnea, agitation
>50	Loss of consciousness, seizures, coma, death

Interventions

1. Provide 100% oxygen via mask until levels are below 10–20%

Electrical Injury

The electrical current enters through the skin, converts to heat, passes through the body, and exits the body—thus producing entrance and exit burn wounds. Although the external burn wounds may appear minor, the notable injury occurs internally along the path created by the current, between the entrance and exit wounds.

Assessment

1. Determine the following:
   - Δ path of the current
   - Δ duration of contact
   - Δ intensity and type of current
     - low voltage
     - high voltage
     - alternating current
     - direct current
   - Δ resistance of the tissues to the passage of current
2. Evaluate entrance/exit wounds

Interventions (in addition to previously discussed care)

1. Maintain ABCs
2. Obtain cardiac enzymes
3. Obtain 12 lead EKG
4. Continue cardiac monitoring

Chemical Injury

Assessment

1. Determine the following:
   - Δ type of chemical
   - Δ concentration
   - Δ duration of contact
   - Δ mechanism of injury
   - Δ extent of tissue penetration

Interventions

1. Remove clothing from patient.
2. Lavage area with copious amount of water or saline:
    Δ 30 minutes for acid burns
    Δ 1–2 hours for alkaline burns

POSSIBLE CERVICAL SPINE INJURY
(CONSIDER POSSIBILITY OF NECK INJURY
WITH ANY OTHER INJURY)

Assessment

A. Obtain and record basic triage assessment that includes:
1. mechanism of injury
2. alteration in range of motion (do not test range of motion [ROM] of neck)
3. alteration in sensory perception

Interventions

1. For patients presenting ambulatory to the ED, and there is an indication that a neck injury may have occurred, prepare for immediate immobilization of the patient's c-spine.
   Δ Explain the importance of and the procedure for immobilization of the patient's c-spine.
   Δ Obtain the correct size collar for the patient.
   Δ Place collar on patient and secure appropriately.
   Δ Immediately place the patient onto a stretcher (follow specific departmental policy for c-spine immobilization process in triage).
   Δ Contact ED physician if not already involved in care of the patient.
   Δ Clearly document the process of c-spine immobilization.
2. Complete remainder of basic triage assessment and document carefully.
3. Frequently observe and communicate with the patient.
   Δ Place patient in room easily visible and audible from nurse's station.
   Δ Educate patient (and visitors) of the importance of remaining supine on stretcher until c-spine is cleared by physician.
4. Keep patient NPO.
5. Have suction set up and ready for use at bedside.
6. Be prepared to log roll patient:
   • if patient vomits
   • if MD needs assistance with examination of patient's back
7. Undress patient for MD evaluation:
   Δ MAINTAIN C-SPINE IMMOBILIZATION while undressing patient.
   Δ if patient is potentially unstable, cut clothes from patient.
   Δ provide for patient's privacy and warmth
8. Quickly evaluate the possibility of transferring the patient to a trauma center and arrange for an appropriate transfer following hospital policy.

 ALERT If patient is uncooperative, unstable, or at risk of vomiting, RN (or other qualified hospital appointed employee) must remain with patient during procedures and transports.

> ### CHEST PAIN

Facts:

Δ Over 57 million Americans have some sort of cardiovascular disease.
Δ Over 7 million Americans have angina.
Δ At least 250,000 Americans annually die **within 1 hour** of the onset of chest pain (American Heart Association, 1994).

 ALERT   Quick and accurate triage assessment of chest pain is *essential!*

 Assessment

A. Obtain and record triage assessment that includes:
  1. Description of pain
     Δ **P**rovoking factors (what makes it better or worse?)
     Δ **Q**uality of pain
     Δ **R**egion/radiation of pain
     Δ **S**everity of pain (1–10 scale)
     Δ **T**ime (onset, duration, constant/intermittent)
     Δ **T**reatment (what has the patient already tried?)
  2. Associated signs and symptoms including:
     Δ dyspnea (on exertion or positional)
     Δ left shoulder pain
     Δ left arm pain
     Δ syncope
     Δ palpitations
     Δ fatigue
     Δ nausea
     Δ diaphoresis
     Δ indigestion
     Δ dizziness
     Δ cough
     Δ hemoptysis
     Δ headache
     Δ vomiting
     Δ behavioral changes
     Δ back pain
     Δ jaw pain
  3. Associated risk factors
     Δ atherosclerosis
     Δ hypertension

Δ high cholesterol levels
Δ family history of heart disease
Δ children with congenital heart disease
Δ smoking
Δ diabetes
Δ obesity
Δ stress
Δ chemical dependency
Δ alcoholism
Δ lack of exercise
Δ cardiac surgery

Immediate Care If

Δ Male >30 years old
Δ Female >35 years old
Δ History of:
- angina
- myocardial infarction
- thrombolytics
- any associated risk factors
- stroke
- coronary artery disease
- cocaine use within the past 24 hours

Interventions

1. Continue triage assessment while beginning treatment. Obtain vital signs, including:
   Δ blood pressure
   Δ apical heart rate
   Δ respiratory rate
   Δ temperature
   Δ room air oximetry
2. Administer oxygen at 2–4 L/minute with nasal cannula
   Exception: Use 100% oxygen if:
   Δ patient is obviously hypoxic
   Δ room air oximetry is <92%
3. Obtain 12-lead EKG
4. Continue triage if noncardiac chest pain:
   Δ Obtain basic triage assessment per protocol
   Δ Consider other sources of pain, including:
   - respiratory
   - gastrointestinal
   - musculoskeletal

Chest Pain: Causes and Characteristics

System	Cause	Characteristic
Cardio-vascular	Acute Myocardial Infarction	Pain may be described as aching, pressure, squeezing, burning, tightness Intensity: vague to severe Location of pain: substernal, epigastric, between shoulder blades Radiation of pain to neck, jaw, arm, back Diabetic neuropathy patients may have only vague pain Associated signs and symptoms: pallor, ashen skin, diaphoresis, dyspnea, nausea, vomiting
	Aneurysm	Pain may be described as searing, continuous, severe Radiation of pain to back, neck, or shoulder(s) Associated signs and symptoms: hypotension, diaphoresis, syncope
	Angina	Pain may be described as squeezing, pressure, tightness—relieved with rest or nitroglycerin Pain may be persistent or intermittent Occurs with activity, anxiety, sex, heavy meals, smoking, or at rest Associated signs and symptoms: dyspnea, nausea, vomiting, diaphoresis, indigestion
	Pericarditis	Pain may be described as severe, continuous, worse when lying on left side Radiation of pain to shoulder or neck History may include recent cardiac surgery, viral illness, or myocardial infarction
	Tachydysrhythmias	Pain may be described as severe, crushing, or generalized pain over chest Associated signs and symptoms: anxiety, tachycardia, tachypnea, dizziness, impending doom
Gastro-intestinal	Hiatal Hernia	Pain may be described as sharp, over the epigastrium Occurs with heavy meals, bending over, lying down
	Indigestion/Peptic Ulcer	Pain may be described as burning, heartburn, pressure Nonradiating pain, not influenced by activity Occurs with empty stomach (peptic ulcer) and heavy meals (indigestion)
Musculo-skeletal	Costochondritis	Pain may be described as sharp, severe Localized to affected area with tenderness on palpation Associated signs and symptoms: cough, "cold"
	Muscle Strain	Pain may be described as aching Occurs with increased use or exercise of upper body muscles
	Trauma	Pain is severe with localization over area of trauma Pain worsens with palpation, movement, or cough May have dyspnea

continued

Chest Pain: Causes and Characteristics (Continued)

System	Cause	Characteristic
Pulmonary	Noxious Fumes/ Smoke Inhalation	Pain may be described as searing, sense of suffocation, burning
		History includes exposure to fire, pesticide, carbon monoxide, paint, chemicals
		Associated signs and symptoms: dyspnea, hypoxia, cough, pallor, ashen skin, cyanosis, singed nasal hairs, soot in oropharynx, gray or black sputum, hoarseness, drooling
		Carbon monoxide poisoning may additionally show nausea, headache, confusion, dizziness, irritability, decreased judgment, ataxia, collapse
	Pleuritic	May be described as sharp, localized, gradual onset yet pain is continuous
		Pain worsens with breathing, coughing, movement
		Common in smokers
	Pneumonia (parenchymal)	Pain may be described as dull discomfort to severe pain, continuous in nature
		Associated signs and symptoms: fever, shortness of breath, tachycardia, malaise, cough, tachypnea
		Children may complain of *abdominal* pain instead of chest pain
	Pneumothorax	Pain may be described as sudden onset, sharp, severe
		Associated signs and symptoms: acute shortness of breath
	Pulmonary Embolism	Pain may be described as severe, crushing, sudden onset
		Acute shortness of breath
		Risk factors include recent long bone fractures, surgery, smoking, use of oral contraceptives
Other	Anxiety	Pain may be described as aching, stabbing
		Associated with stressful event, anxiety
		Associated signs and symptoms: hyperventilation, carpal spasms, palpitations, weakness, fear, or sense of impending doom

DIFFICULTY BREATHING

Assessment

A. Obtain and record triage assessment:
  1. Ask patient the time of onset of respiratory difficulty.
  2. Assess vital signs for:
     Δ tachypnea
     Δ tachycardia
     Δ bradypnea
     Δ room air oximetry (<90% critical)
  3. Assess for exertional effects due to walking or speaking in full sentences.
  4. Determine associated signs and symptoms:
     Δ pallor
     Δ stridor
     Δ wheezing
     Δ absent breath sounds
     Δ nasal flaring on infants
     Δ cyanosis
     Δ retractions
     Δ crackles
     Δ ashen skin
     Δ use of accessory muscles
     Δ diminished breath sounds
  5. Place patient in respiratory isolation room when presenting with any combination of the following:
     Δ hemoptysis
     Δ fever
     Δ night sweats
     Δ known tuberculosis (TB) history without completed treatment
     Δ profound fatigue
     Δ significant weight loss for no apparent reason
     Δ cough lasting longer than 3 weeks
  6. Obtain past medical history, including any previous pulmonary diseases or injuries.

Immediate Care If

Δ cyanotic
Δ stridorous
Δ drooling
Δ room air oximetry <90%
Δ patient is unable to speak in full sentences

Interventions

1. Assign patient to exam room according to ED protocol (acute vs. nonacute bed)
2. Initiate care as per protocol:
   Δ assist patient to undress fully
   Δ place adult patients on cardiac monitor
   Δ administer oxygen by 50% mask or greater (use care if history of COPD)
   Δ obtain initial, or repeat triage vital signs
   Δ consider saline lock or normal saline IV at KVO rate per ED (protocol)
   Δ consider drawing lab samples per ED protocol
3. Notify ED physician of patient status
4. Utilize appropriate flow sheet for **documentation** purposes as necessary

■ PEAK FLOW MEASUREMENT

Many indicators are assessed during the evaluation and treatment of patients with respiratory difficulty. Measurement of the patient's peak end-expiratory flow volume may be useful in establishing the severity of the patient's crisis and is helpful in providing a baseline understanding of the patient's respiratory status.

Peak flow readings are usually performed on patients during their initial assessment and after each nebulizer treatment. This process may be individualized to meet the treating physician's preference or the patient's ability to comply.

INSTRUCTIONS FOR USE

1. It is preferable to perform this test while the patient is standing. If the patient's condition does not permit this, then all peak flow measurements during this ED visit should be done with the patient in the same position.
2. Have the patient hold the peak flow meter lightly, making sure the fingers do not obstruct the slot or interfere with the movement of the marker.
3. Have the patient take in as deep a breath as possible.
4. Place the mouthpiece in the patient's mouth, and instruct him or her to seal the lips firmly around the outside of the mouthpiece.
5. Have the patient blow as hard and as fast as possible into the mouthpiece. This action is best described as a hard "huff."
6. The marker will move up the scale. Read the value.
7. Return the marker to the lower end of the scale.
8. Repeat the test twice more, and document the best of the three readings.

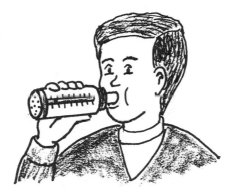

Peak flow measurement.

Predicted Average Peak Expiratory Flow (L/min): Pediatric Patients

Height (Inches)	Values (Male or Female)
43	147
44	160
45	173
46	187
47	200
48	214
49	227
50	240
51	254
52	267
53	280
54	293
55	307
56	320
57	334
58	347
59	360
60	373
61	387
62	400
63	413
64	427
65	440
66	454

Predicted Average Peak Expiratory Flow (L/min): Males

Age	Height (Inches)				
	60	65	70	75	80
20	554	602	649	693	740
25	543	590	636	679	725
30	532	577	622	664	710
35	521	565	609	651	695
40	509	552	596	636	680
45	498	540	583	622	665
50	486	527	569	607	649
55	475	515	556	593	634
60	463	502	542	578	618
65	452	490	529	564	603
70	440	477	515	550	587

Predicted Average Peak Expiratory Flow (L/min): Females

Age	Height (Inches)				
	55	60	65	70	75
20	390	423	460	496	529
25	385	418	454	490	523
30	380	413	448	483	516
35	375	408	442	476	509
40	370	402	436	470	502
45	365	397	430	464	495
50	360	391	424	457	448
55	355	386	418	451	482
60	350	380	412	445	475
65	345	375	406	439	468
70	340	369	400	432	461

DOMESTIC VIOLENCE: CHILD ABUSE
AND ELDER ABUSE

Domestic violence includes all instances of violent behavior toward persons living permanently or frequently within the same household and the abuse or neglect of children or elders.

Assessment

A. Perform basic triage assessment per protocol.
B. Identify and document possibility or reality of domestic violence, elder abuse/neglect or child abuse or neglect.
    Δ Patient admits to history of injury by family member or friend.
    Δ History conflicts or is inconsistent with injuries.
    Δ Suspicion of domestic violence raised by emergency medical services or other third party
    Δ Known previous history of domestic violence
    Δ Unexplained delay in seeking treatment
    Δ Patient fearful of household member or reluctant to respond when questioned
    Δ Patient exhibits poor personal hygiene and/or inappropriate clothing
    Δ Household member:
- oversolicitous
- angy or indifferent toward patient
- prevents the patient from interacting privately or speaking openly
- refuses to provide necessary assistance
- refuses or hesitates to permit transfer to hospital
- is concerned about minor patient problem but not with the patient's serious health issue(s)

    Δ Patient exhibits injuries suggestive of nonaccidental etiology:
- cigarette or other burns
- strap marks
- multiple bruises
- human bite marks
- long bone fractures in infants and young children
- injuries involving cheeks, ears, torso, buttocks, genitalia

    Δ Parents leave injured or sick child alone in ED while they:
- go to the cafeteria
- have a cigarette
- use the telephone

C. If triage nurse suspects the possibility of domestic violence, arrange to interview patient privately, and consider asking:
1. "Have you ever been hit, slapped, kicked, or otherwise physically hurt by someone close to you?"
    Δ If the answer is *yes,* ask the date of the last episode.
2. "Have you ever been forced to have sexual activities?"
    Δ If the answer is *yes,* ask the date of the last episode (McFarlane, 1995).

3. If the triage nurse suspects the possibility of child or elder abuse, ask the parents or caretaker at various times throughout the patient's stay in the ED:
   Δ "Tell me again, how did this happen?"
     • the ED staff will often be able to pick up inconsistencies in the history if abuse has occurred (Miller, 1996).

ALERT   For all pediatric and elder patients who present with *any* injury, appropriate assessment for the possibility of abuse or neglect should occur. Consider an easy documentation tool, such as the sample Pediatric Injury Assessment form or the Elder Abuse form.

D. Complete remainder of basic triage assessment per protocol.

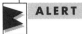

Immediate Care If

Δ Patient has serious injuries or is in danger.
(Separate the adult patient from family/care taker/significant other if possibility of assault, abuse, or neglect occurred.)

ALERT   **Refer to your department's policy for specific procedural information regarding the notification of:**

   Δ law enforcement agency
   Δ child abuse hotline
   Δ adult protective service
   Δ rape crisis advocate

Carefully document:

   Δ Triage assessment
   Δ Detailed history/indication of any information related to the possibility of:
     • domestic violence
     • elder abuse/neglect
     • child abuse/neglect
   Δ Only that information that is pertinent to the *medical treatment* of the patient

Do not attempt to document for the *legal treatment* of your patient. That should be left to the law enforcement agency and the district attorney's office.

Bruise Assessment

Color of Bruise	Age of Bruise
Red Reddish blue	Less than 24 hours since time of injury
Dark blue Dark purple	1–4 days
Green Yellow-green	5–7 days
Yellow Brown	7–10 days
Normal tint Disappearance of bruise	1–3 weeks

■ DOCUMENTATION OF PEDIATRIC AND ELDER INJURIES

Nurses must always be alert for the possibility of abuse or neglect when triaging. Because a busy nurse can easily overlook subtle abuse injuries, departments should have a system in place that ensures that each injury suffered by a patient is adequately evaluated for the possibility of abuse or neglect.

The following pages are sample documentation tools that have been created specifically for use in the triage setting and can be accurately completed in a matter of seconds. This provides appropriate evaluation of each patient situation as well as proper documentation of the assessment. If after completing this quick evaluation tool, abuse is suspected, a more comprehensive tool on the back of the form can be used for an in-depth assessment and documentation of this child and follow-up.

INSTRUCTIONS FOR USING THE FORM

1. Fill out the demographic information on the top. For departments that use address-o-graph machines, a space has been provided at the upper right of the form.
2. While obtaining the triage history, the nurse will check off the appropriate answer for each of the boxed questions. For most non-abuse type injuries, each answer will be "no."
3. If an answer is "yes," a clarifying comment must be made in the box to the right.
4. If suspicion of child abuse is present upon completing the front of the form, the health care team should proceed to the back of the form as necessary.
5. This form should be used as a complement to the regular departmental documentation tools, not instead of them.

PATIENT NAME _____

PEDIATRIC INJURY ASSESSMENT FORM

FOR USE IN ALL CHILDREN LESS THAN 18 YEARS OF AGE WITH:

- INJURIES
- EXPOSURES
- SUSPICIOUS ILLNESSES

DATE: _____ CHILD'S AGE: _____

WHERE DID INJURY OCCUR? _____

HISTORY PROVIDED BY: _____

HISTORY OF EVENT: _____

PERSON(S) SUPERVISING CHILD WHEN EVENT OCCURRED: _____

HIGH-RISK INDICATORS FOR POSSIBLE CHILD ABUSE/NEGLECT	YES	NO	N/A	COMMENTS
Are findings inconsistent with history based on age and development of child?				
Did caretaker delay in obtaining medical care?				
Was there an unexplained absence of supervision at the time of injury?				
Is the appearance/hygiene of parent(s) inappropriate for circumstances?				
Is behavior of child inappropriate?				
Is there evidence of substance abuse?				
Is the injury a suspicious burn or human bite?				
Are there any signs of shaken baby syndrome?				
Does the injury involve the cheeks, ears, neck, chest, back, abdomen, buttocks or genitalia?				
Are there any long bone fractures?				
Are there inconsistencies or changes in the history?				

If the answer to any of the above questions is "yes", explain under "comments."

If suspicion of child abuse for these or any other reasons exists, proceed to the next page.

Signatures _____ RN _____ MD

					DESCRIPTION OF INJURY(S)		
INJURY NUMBER	TYPE OF INJURY	SHAPE	SIZE	COLOR	ESTIMATED AGE OF INJURY	STATED AGE OF INJURY	EXPLANATION BY: MOTHER, FATHER, CHILD, BABY-SITTER, OTHER
1							
2							
3							
4							
5							

The investigation of child abuse may include contact with the following individuals/agencies:

1. Pediatrician _____ _____ _____
   NAME   TIME   COMMENTS
                     CONTACTED

2. Child Protective Services _____ _____ _____
   NAME   TIME   COMMENTS
                     CONTACTED

3. Law Enforcement _____ _____ _____
   * Must be contacted if AGENCY TIME COMMENTS
   immediate intervention CONTACTED
   is needed

4. Child Abuse Hotline _____ _____ _____
   AGENCY   TIME   COMMENTS
                     CONTACTED

5. Photographs Taken?   Yes ☐   No ☐

6. Was Child Admitted?   Yes ☐   No ☐

7. If child was not admitted, describe disposition: _____
_____
_____

Signatures _____ RN _____ MD

PATIENT NAME _____

ELDER ABUSE ASSESSMENT FORM

FOR USE WITH ANY ELDER PERSON PRESENTING WITH:

- INJURIES
- EXPOSURES
- SUSPICIOUS ILLNESSES

DATE: _____ PATIENT'S AGE: _____

HISTORY PROVIDED BY: _____

HISTORY OF EVENT: _____

PERSON(S) WITH PATIENT WHEN EVENT OCCURRED: _____

NORMAL BEHAVIORS OF PATIENT

☐ confused ☐ aggressive ☐ memory loss
☐ disoriented ☐ wandering ☐ altered judgement

HIGH-RISK INDICATORS FOR POSSIBLE ELDER ABUSE/NEGLECT	YES	NO	N/A	COMMENTS
Are findings inconsistent with history?				
Did patient/caretaker delay in obtaining medical care?				
Is the appearance/hygiene of patient inappropriate for circumstances?				
Is behavior of patient/caretaker inappropriate?				
Any unusual bruising patterns?				
Is the injury a suspicious burn or human bite?				
Does the injury involve the cheeks, ears, neck, chest, back, abdomen, buttocks, genitalia, wrists, or ankles?				
Is there evidence of failure to provide food, clothing, shelter, medications, supervision, etc.?				
Is there evidence of verbal, mental, sexual, financial, or substance abuse?				
Are there inconsistencies or changes in the history?				

If the answer to any of the above questions is "yes", explain under "comments."

If suspicion of elder abuse for these or any other reasons exists, proceed to the next page.

Signatures _____ RN _____ MD

DESCRIPTION OF INJURY(S)							
INJURY NUMBER	TYPE OF INJURY	SHAPE	SIZE	COLOR	ESTIMATED AGE OF INJURY	STATED AGE OF INJURY	EXPLANATION GIVEN BY:
1							
2							
3							
4							
5							

The investigation of elder abuse may include contact with the following individuals/agencies:

1. Primary Care Provider _____   _____   _____
                                 NAME   TIME CONTACTED   COMMENTS

2. Adult Protective Services _____   _____   _____
                                 NAME   TIME CONTACTED   COMMENTS

3. Law Enforcement _____   _____   _____
     * Must be contacted if   AGENCY   TIME   COMMENTS
       immediate intervention   CONTACTED
       is needed

4. Photographs Taken?   Yes ☐   No ☐

5. Was Patient Admitted?   Yes ☐   No ☐

6. If patient was not admitted, describe disposition: _____
_____
_____

7. Comments: _____
_____
_____

Signatures _____ RN _____ MD

ENDOCRINE EMERGENCIES

The endocrine system is a complex one that works closely with other regulatory systems of the body. It is composed of many secretory glands, with the primary function of maintaining homeostasis within the body and regulating metabolism.

Assessment

A. Perform basic triage assessment per protocol.

> **ALERT** Intervene *immediately* if a life-threatening situation is discovered.

Hypoglycemia

Serum glucose <50 mg/dl in adults, <60 mg/dl in children

Assessment

1. Common signs:
   - △ tachycardia
   - △ restlessness
   - △ palpitations
   - △ cool, diaphoretic skin
   - △ anxiety
   - △ tremors
   - △ irritability
2. Neurologic deficit signs:
   - △ headache
   - △ slurred speech
   - △ diplopia
   - △ seizures
   - △ confusion
   - △ combativeness
   - △ blurred vision
   - △ coma

Interventions

1. Administer oral glucose to adult who is awake, alert, and has a gag reflex.
2. Administer 50–100 cc of 50% Dextrose IV push to adult who is semiconscious/nonresponsive).
3. Administer 1–2 mg/Kg of 25% Dextrose IV push to child who is unconscious.

ALERT *Never use 50% dextrose for children, as it will cause vein necrosis.*

Diabetic Ketoacidosis (DKA)

Assessment

1. Gradual onset (3–7 days) of symptoms:
   Δ polyuria
   Δ polydipsia
   Δ weakness
   Δ polyphagia
   Δ vomiting
   Δ fever
   Δ lethargy
   Δ abdominal pain
2. Objective signs:
   Δ hypotension
   Δ tachycardia
   Δ acetone breath
   Δ decreased mental status
   Δ Kussmaul's breathing
   Δ hot, dry skin with poor turgor
3. Laboratory values:
   Δ serum glucose >300 mg/dl
   Δ decreased serum bicarbonate
   Δ elevated acetone level
   Δ decreased arterial pH
   Δ elevated blood urea nitrogen (BUN) and creatinine
   Δ elevated hemoglobin and hematocrit
   Δ potassium level quickly fluctuates as treatment progresses

Interventions

1. Rapidly identify DKA.
2. Continually reassess and treat with fluids, electrolytes, and insulin administration.

Hyperglycemic Hyperosmolar Nonketotic Coma (HHNC)

Assessment

1. Slow onset (10–14 days) of symptoms:
   Δ polyuria
   Δ polydipsia
   Δ fever
2. Objective signs:
   Δ tachycardia
   Δ aphasia
   Δ hypotension
   Δ tremors
   Δ hyperreflexia
   Δ severe dehydration
   Δ decreased mental status
     • from confused to unresponsive
   Δ nuchal rigidity
   Δ focal seizures
3. Laboratory values:
   Δ serum glucose >800–1000 mg/dl
   Δ serum osmolality >350 mOsm/Kg
   Δ decreased serum sodium level
   Δ decreased potassium level
   Δ elevated BUN
   Δ elevated hematocrit
   Δ elevated creatinine

Interventions

1. Maintain ABCs.
2. Continually monitor vital signs and fluid status carefully and precisely.
3. Replace fluid deficit slowly to prevent cerebral edema (may be 8–12 L).
4. Closely monitor and correct electrolyte imbalances.

Adrenal Gland Emergency: Addisonian Crisis

Assessment

1. Common signs:
   Δ nausea
   Δ vomiting
   Δ weakness
   Δ lethargy
   Δ hyperpigmentation
   Δ hypotension (not responsive to IV fluid bolus)
   Δ fatigue
   Δ anorexia
   Δ weight loss
   Δ abdominal pain
2. Less common signs:
   Δ diarrhea
   Δ delirium
   Δ constipation
   Δ increased motor activity

Interventions

1. Continually, monitor cardiovascular and fluid volume status carefully.
2. Correct fluid volume deficit (usually about 3L). Aggressive replacement of fluid is necessary.
3. Administer corticosteroids, as necessary.
4. Correct hypoglycemia, as indicated.

EYE INJURIES

Assessment

A. Obtain and record triage assessment that includes:
   1. Onset of problem (acute vs. gradual)
   2. Known precipitating event (exposure to splash or fumes, head injury, etc.)
      Δ Was protective eye wear being worn?
      Δ When was the injury?
      Δ Was any care given at time of injury (rinse, patch, etc.)?
   3. Appearance of both eyes.
      Δ infection (pain, discharged, redness, edema, periorbital warmth)
      Δ foreign body
      Δ photophobic
      Δ hyphema
      Δ deformity or irregularity of the eye
      Δ no obvious signs of problem
   4. Visual acuity (refer to Snellen chart later in manual)—obtain during triage assessment, and again after treatment
B. Assess blunt or sharp trauma for:
      Δ object causing injury (tennis ball, stick, etc.)
      Δ object size and composition
      Δ velocity of force
      Δ direction of force onto eye
C. Assess arc burns for:
   (Arc burns occur from unprotected exposure of the eye to welding devices.)
      Δ time since exposure
      Δ distance from flame
      Δ duration of exposure
D. Assess chemical splash for:
      Δ chemical name(s) (Call poison control if chemical identification necessary.)
      Δ initial eye symptoms/current symptoms
      Δ irrigation substance and duration of irrigation

Immediate Care If

Δ Penetrating injury to the eye
Δ Chemical splash injury

Interventions

1. If in a penetrating injury, the foreign body is visible:
   Δ stabilize the area surrounding the object
   Δ avoid any movement of, or contact with, the foreign body.

2. If in a penetrating injury the foreign body is already removed, place a dry sterile patch over the eye and review patient status with the ED physician.
3. With a chemical splash injury:
   Δ Test pH of eye
   Δ Review patient status with ED physician
   Λ Prepare for:
   - possible instillation of two drops of eye anesthetic in affected eye
   - flush upper and lower conjunctival fornix with direct stream of 1000 cc normal saline
4. Complete remainder of basic triage assessment per protocol, and carefully document all information obtained during the triage assessment.

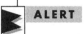

ALERT   Patients with eye injuries may have visual difficulties, especially depth perception. Protect for their safety while walking, and use side rails when they are in bed. Continual patient education is crucial to allay heightened patient anxiety.

■ SNELLEN CHART FOR VISUAL ACUITY

The purpose of using the Snellen eye chart when triaging is to assess any changes in the patient's normal vision. If the patient normally wears corrective lenses for distance, then he or she should wear them during the assessment of visual acuity.

Testing for visual acuity *must* be done both before and after treatment of the patient's eye problem. This illustrates the patient's baseline on arriving to the ED and also reassesses the patient's acuity after the treatment is complete to document any improvement and to show that no harm was done by the treatment.

The results of this test are documented in the form of a fraction. The numerator is the distance the patient is standing from the chart (20 ft). The denominator, which is listed by each line of the chart, represents the distance at which the average eye can read that particular line of the chart.

TO PERFORM A VISUAL ACUITY TEST

1. Have the patient stand 20 feet away from the Snellen chart.
2. Instruct the patient to cover the *unaffected* eye.
3. Have the patient read the letters starting at the top of the chart, using only the affected eye (you always want the patient to read with the "bad" eye first).
4. Record the last line of which the patient can read at least 50% of the letters, indicating how many were missed (e.g., right eye 20/40, -2)
5. Repeat this by covering affected eye, having the patient perform the test with the unaffected eye, and document the results.
6. Repeat this one last time, having the patient use both eyes to read the chart.

Documentation of results for the visual acuity testing should be recorded for each eye and for both eyes, should indicate if the patient used corrective lenses, and should indicate the time performed.
For example:

1945: With glasses: right eye (OD) 20/30, -2
                    left eye (OS)   20/20, -0
                    both eyes (OU) 20/20, -0

FACIAL, DENTAL, AND EAR/NOSE/THROAT (ENT) INJURIES

ALERT *Verify airway patency prior to and along with the assessment of these injuries. Consider possibility of c-spine or brain injury.*

Assessment

A. Obtain and record triage assessment that includes:
- Δ Nature of injury:
  - blunt
  - burn
  - blast
  - crush
  - penetrating
- Δ Mechanism of injury:
  - size
  - direction
  - velocity
- Δ Contributing factors:
  - caliber of weapon
  - height of fall
  - damage to car
- Δ Time of injury
- Δ Pain:
  - quality
  - location
- Δ Parethesia
- Δ Immediate care of injured area

B. Utilize universal precautions during assessment progression
- Δ Face:
  - skin integrity
  - bleeding
  - wound size
  - soft tissue swelling
  - wound location
- Δ Scalp:
  - inspect and palpate for deformities or wounds
- Δ Facial structures:
  - symmetry
  - elongation of midface

- depression of bony structures
- downward displacement of globe of eye

Δ Visual acuity:
- perform for any injury involving the eye(s) or adjacent areas

Δ Palpate zygomas and bony orbits:
- swelling
- deformity
- point tenderness

Δ Ear and mastoid areas:
- lacerations
- drainage
- ecchymosis (Battle's sign)

Δ Nose
- alignment
- septal hematoma
- deformity
- epistaxis
- swelling

Δ Maxilla
- pain
- ecchymosis
- malocclusion
- periorbital swelling
- midface mobility

Δ Teeth: Using gloved finger, palpate for:
- fractures
- subluxations
- avulsions

Δ Jaw occlusion (bite):
- pain
- malalignment
- range of motion

C. Complete remainder of triage protocol, and document carefully. Up to 25% of all significant facial injuries eventually result in litigation. Consider drawings and photographs for the medical record (Kitt, 1995).

 Interventions

1. Continue to assess the airway patency because the patient is at risk of developing airway compromise due to:
   Δ nasal and intraoral bleeding
   Δ fractured teeth
   Δ vomitus
   Δ secretions

    Δ pharyngeal hematomas

    Δ tongue displacement

    Δ edema

    Δ foreign bodies

    Δ altered level of consciousness

2. Apply ice to facial injury to minimize swelling
3. Avulsed teeth should be:

    Δ handled by the crown only

    Δ placed in normal saline, milk, or saliva until reimplantation occurs

    Δ Sav-A-Tooth is an acceptable preservative and is sold over the counter (OTC)

4. Administer dT per departmental protocol
5. Perform Halo test on nasal and ear drainage, checking for CSF leak

FEBRILE CHILD

Assessment

A. Obtain and record triage assessment:
   1. Fever
      Δ onset
      Δ duration
      Δ degree
      Δ route
   2. Associated symptoms and behavior
      Δ irritability, change in normal play behavior, lethargy
      Δ feeding problems
      Δ abnormal cry
      Δ seizure
      Δ respiratory symptoms
      Δ rash
      Δ change in urination or stooling
      Δ tugging at ears
      Δ limping or refusal to use an extremity
      Δ cough
      Δ localized swelling or erythema
      Δ vomiting
   3. Use of antipyretics, including:
      Δ type
      Δ time of last dose
      Δ amount administered
   4. Immunization status on chart per ED protocol
B. Obtain and record vital signs.
      Δ Respirations:
         • must be counted for a full 60-second period on children <1 year old
         • document if child was crying, sleeping, etc.
      Δ Heart Rate:
         • apical pulse on children <3 years old
           (caution using heart rate reading from automatic BP machines)
      Δ Temperature:
         • follow facility policy on route of temperature
         • recommend rectal temperature on all children <5 years old with suspicion of febrile illness
      Δ Room air oximetry:
         • may need assistance from respiratory therapy (critical reading <90%)
      Δ Blood pressure:
         • obtain after all other vital signs have been obtained
         • omit if child <5 years old and patient agitation could compromise patient's condition

Immediate Care If

Δ Patient is <12 weeks of age and rectal temperature >100.4°F as recorded by ED staff or reported by parent within the past 6 hours.

Δ Rectal temperature <96°F as recorded by ED staff or reported by parent within the past 6 hours.

Δ Seizure, difficulty breathing, acute onset of skin rash, or any general discomfort on the part of the triage nurse.

ALERT   Notify the ED physician immediately if any of the above occurs!

Interventions

1. Undress completely, down to diaper or panties
2. Wrap in blanket if necessary
3. Administer acetaminophen/ibuprofen per department protocol
4. Administer oxygen if:
   Δ respiratory rate elevated for age
   Δ room air oximetry <90%

GYNECOLOGICAL ISSUES

Women seek health care for a variety of reasons from an ED or urgent care setting. Many reasons involve the female reproductive system. The triage nurse must possess excellent clinical assessment skills as well as sensitivity to the psychological needs of a woman in need of gynecological care. Women may present with any of the following:

Δ fever
Δ fatigue
Δ nausea
Δ vaginal bleeding
Δ dyspareunia
Δ trauma
Δ abdominal pain
Δ dysuria
Δ vomiting
Δ purulent vaginal discharge
Δ dysmenorrhea
Δ sexual assault

 ALERT Sexual assault survivors are assigned a high priority and escorted directly into a private room.

General Issues

 Assessment

A. Obtain basic triage assessment per protocol.
B. Perform abdominal pain triage assessment as necessary.

Bartholinitis

Infection or inflammation of Bartholin's glands, which lie on both sides of the vagina at the base of the labia minora.

 Assessment

1. Common symptoms:
   Δ pain (moderate to severe)
   Δ swelling
   Δ tenderness

Δ cellulitis
Δ erythema
Δ edema
2. Laboratory values:
Δ possible culture for organism

Interventions

1. Assist with incision and drainage of gland if indicated.
2. Administer antibiotic therapy as prescribed.
3. Provide patient education, including:
Δ sitz baths three to four times a day
Δ STD transmission and available precautions
Δ infection or abscess may recur

Herpes Genitalis (Herpes Simplex Virus Type 2)

Viral infection that causes lesions on the cervix, vagina, and external genitalia.

Assessment

1. Common symptoms:
Δ painful lesions
Δ fever
Δ pruritus
Δ inguinal tenderness
Δ erythema
Δ watery discharge from vagina or urethra
Δ dyspareunia
Δ malaise
Δ dysuria
Δ lymphadenopathy
Δ bleeding
2. Clinical manifestations:
Δ Lesions occur 2–10 days after initial exposure and last 3–6 weeks.
Δ First manifestation is the most severe and prolonged.
Δ Lesions may proceed from macules → papules → vesicles → pustules → ulcers, which may crust and heal with scars.
Δ Lesions usually present as multiple vesicles with a clear, shiny, or red base.
Δ Lesions are usually located on the
• vagina
• perineal area

- cervix
- vulva
- buttocks
- thighs

 Interventions

1. Serology for syphilis
2. Administer acyclovir (or other antiviral agents) to decrease:
   Δ pain
   Δ length of infection
   Δ healing time
3. Provide patient education, including:
   Δ complete information on herpes genitalis, including care of lesions
   Δ STD transmission and available precautions
   Δ HIV counseling and testing

Pelvic Inflammatory Disease (PID)

Acute or chronic infection that involves the fallopian tubes, ovaries, uterus, pelvic peritoneum, or pelvic connective tissue.

 Assessment

1. History:
   Δ new sexual partner within past 2 months
   Δ multiple sexual partners
   Δ early onset of sexual activity
   Δ use of intrauterine devices
   Δ surgical procedures
2. Common symptoms:
   Δ fever
   Δ pelvic or abdominal pain
   Δ purulent vaginal discharge
   Δ irregular menstrual bleeding
   Δ dyspareunia
   Δ dysuria or urinary frequency
   Δ walking worsens abdominal pain (walks hunched forward)
   Δ cervical motion tenderness during pelvic exam
3. Laboratory values:
   Δ elevated white blood cell count
   Δ pregnancy test

△ serology for syphilis
△ elevated sedimentation rates
△ cervical cultures to isolate organisms

 Interventions

1. Administer antibiotic therapy as per current recommendations.
2. Provide patient education, including:
   △ early signs/symptoms of PID
   △ STD transmission and available precautions
   △ treatment of partner(s)
   △ HIV counseling and testing

Vaginitis

Vaginal inflammation caused by the introduction of pathogens or irritants.

 Assessment

1. History:
   △ nature of vaginal discharge
   △ past illnesses or STDs
   △ medications being used
   △ vaginal hygiene practices
2. Common symptoms:
   △ dysuria
   △ dyspareunia
   △ pelvic pain
   △ vaginal discharge (color, character)
   △ perineal
     • itching
     • burning
     • irritation
     • odor
3. Types of vaginitis:
   △ Simple vaginitis (contact vaginitis)
     • caused by poor hygiene, contact allergens, foreign bodies
     • increased vaginal discharge with itching, edema, burning, redness
     • treated by discontinuance of causative agent
   △ Gardnerella vaginitis (nonspecific or bacterial)
     • caused by an organism other than Trichomonas, Candida, or Gonorrhea
     • may or may not be considered a sexually transmitted disease
     • vaginal discharge with a fishy odor when exposed to potassium hydroxide (KOH)

Δ Trichomonas vaginitis
- copious malodorous discharge, frothy and yellow-green in color
- may have vulvar edema and/or dysuria
- red, speckled punctate hemorrhages on the cervix
- treated with metronidazole (Flagyl) (contraindicated in first trimester of pregnancy)
- partner(s) must be treated with Flagyl to prevent reinfection

Δ Candida albicans (fungal infection)
- caused by use of antibiotics, steroids, douches, oral contraceptives
- frequently associated with pregnancy, obesity, diabetes mellitus, chronic illnesses
- vaginal discharge is thick, irritating, white/yellow color, cheese-like
- may cause itching, dysuria, burning, dyspareunia
- treat with antifungal agents

4. Other:
Δ Human papillomavirus
- causes condyloma acuminatum (venereal warts)
- highly contagious, sexually transmitted disease
- implicated in intraepithelial neoplasia of the vulva, vagina, and cervix
- topical treatment including laser, cryotherapy, electrocautery
- counseling and testing for syphilis, HIV, other STDs

HEADACHE

Assessment

A. Obtain and record triage assessment that includes:
  1. Pain characteristics
     - Δ **P**rovoking factors (what makes it better or worse?)
     - Δ **Q**uality of pain
     - Δ **R**egion/Radiation
     - Δ **S**everity of pain (1–10 scale)
     - Δ **T**ime (onset or duration)
     - Δ **T**reatment
  2. Associated symptoms
     - Δ fever
     - Δ vomiting
     - Δ syncope
     - Δ seizure
     - Δ nausea
     - Δ lethargy
     - Δ visual changes
     - Δ personality changes
     - Δ rash (especially petechial)
     - Δ change in patient's baseline vital signs
     - Δ change in pupil size, equality, or reaction to light
  3. History of:
     - Δ trauma
     - Δ similar headaches
     - Δ exposure to:
       - fumes
       - smoke
       - chemicals
  4. Current treatment
  5. Use of anticoagulants
B. Complete basic triage assessment per protocol, and *document* findings carefully.

Immediate Care If

- Δ Patient states "worst headache of my life"
- Δ Associated fever, stiff neck, or focal signs
- Δ History of recent head trauma
- Δ Systolic BP >180
- Δ Diastolic BP >115
- Δ Warning signs of stroke
  - weakness/numbness in the face, arm, or leg

- visual changes (especially unilateral)
  * sudden dimness
  * blurring
  * decreased visual acuity
- speech disturbance
  * difficulty speaking
  * difficulty understanding speech
- unexplained
  * dizziness
  * vertigo
  * decreased coordination
- sudden, severe headache

Headache Characteristics

Headache	Characteristics

Cerebellar Hemorrhage	<ul><li>Pain
	  * moderate to severe headache</li><li>Associated signs and symptoms
	  * confusion
	  * vomiting
	  * altered gait</li></ul>

Cluster Headaches	<ul><li>Pain
	  * very painful
	  * knifelike
	  * unilateral
	  * over the eye</li><li>Associated signs and symptoms
	  * excessive tearing
	  * facial swelling
	  * redness of the eye
	  * diaphoresis</li></ul>

Increased Intracranial Pressure	<ul><li>Pain
	  * usually not excruciating</li><li>Associated signs and symptoms
	  * nausea or vomiting
	  * lethargy
	  * diplopia
	  * transient visual difficulty</li></ul>

continued

Headache Characteristics (Continued)

Headache	Characteristics

Meningitis	• Pain
	  * mild to severe headache
	  * neck pain or stiffness
	• Associated signs and symptoms
	  * fever
	  * malaise
	  * decreased appetite
	  * irritable

Migraines	• Pain
	  * periodic with gradual onset
	  * throbbing, severe
	  * frequently unilateral, may progress to bilateral
	  * often above of the eye(s)
	• Associated signs and symptoms
	  * photophobia
	  * sensitivity to sound
	  * nausea
	  * vomiting

Sinus Headache	• Pain
	  * over the sinus areas (above the eyes, beside the nose, over the cheekbone)
	• Associated signs and symptoms
	  * fever
	  * nasal drainage or congestion
	  * ear pain
	  * tenderness, swelling or erythema of the sinus area

Subarachnoid Hemorrhage	• Pain
	  * "Worst headache of my life"
	• Associated signs and symptoms
	  * With or without transient impairment of consciousness

Tension	• Pain
	  * Diffuse yet steady dull pain or pressure
	  * "Bandlike" (back of head and neck, across forehead, and/or temporal areas)

HEMATOLOGIC EMERGENCIES

Typically, patients who present to the ED with hematologic emergencies have been previously diagnosed with blood disorders. They should be considered life-threatening episodes, whether they are acute events or exacerbations of a chronic disorder.

General Issues

 Assessment

A. Obtain basic triage assessment per protocol.
B. For both chronic and acute presentations, assess patients for:
  1. Common symptoms:
     Δ weakness
     Δ syncope
     Δ fatigue
     Δ exertional dyspnea
     Δ dizziness
     Δ headache
     Δ fever
  2. Skin changes:
     Δ color
     Δ texture
     Δ petechiae
     Δ moisture
     Δ cyanosis
     Δ ecchymosis
     Δ turgor
     Δ temperature
     Δ jaundice
     Δ pallor
  3. Associated factors:
     Δ precipitating event
     Δ bleeding tendencies
     Δ aggravating or alleviating factors
     Δ joint or muscle
       • redness
       • swelling
       • decreased range of motion
     Δ symptoms
       • onset
       • nature
       • severity
       • duration

Sickle Cell Anemia

This occurs primarily in African Americans and persons of Mediterranean descent.

 Assessment

1. Common precipitating events:
   Δ infection
   Δ depression
   Δ dehydration
   Δ exposure to cold environment
   Δ fever
   Δ hypoxemia
   Δ anxiety
2. Common symptoms:
   Δ fever
   Δ erythema
   Δ organomegaly
   Δ jaundice
   Δ soft tissue swelling
   Δ severe, acute onset of pain
   Δ dehydration
   Δ inflamed joints
   Δ localized warmth
   Δ pallor
3. Laboratory values:
   Δ chronic anemia
   Δ elevated bilirubin count
   Δ reticulocyte count of 5–30%
   Δ variable platelet count
   Δ elevated white blood cell count

 Interventions

1. Maintain ABCs
2. Administer oxygen
3. Insert intravenous access for:
   Δ fluids
   Δ medications
   Δ blood products

ALERT Be *alert* for possible complications, including:
Δ cardiac and renal failure
Δ infarcts to brain, kidneys, lungs
Δ aplastic or sequestrative crisis
Δ infection and sepsis
Δ severe dehydration

Hemophilia

This is characterized by excessive, prolonged, or delayed internal or external bleeding from inherited coagulation disorders, usually occurring only in males.

Assessment

1. Hemarthroses (bleeding into the joint):
   Δ common sites:
   - knee
   - shoulder
   - hip
   - ankle
   - elbow
   - wrist
   Δ common signs and symptoms:
   - pain
   - swelling
   - localized warmth
   - decreased range of motion
2. Intramuscular bleeding:
   Δ common sites:
   - thigh
   - calf
   - forearm
   - iliopsoas (abdomen)
3. Other areas of bleeding:
   Δ common sites:
   - oral cavity
   - intracranial
   - genitourinary
   - gastrointestinal
4. Laboratory values:
   Δ normal or elevated platelet count
   Δ normal or abnormal prothrombin time (PT)

Δ prolonged partial thromboplastin time (PTT)

Δ normal or abnormal bleeding time

 Interventions

1. Maintain ABCs
2. Achieve rapid hemostasis
3. Insert intravenous access for:
   Δ fluids
   Δ medications
   Δ blood products
   Δ factor replacement
4. Treat affected extremity with:
   Δ ice
   Δ elevation
   Δ immobilization
5. Minimize number of venipunctures
6. Always use small-gauge needles.

△ Confidential, nonjudgmental atmosphere is essential when interviewing a patient.
△ The patient may fear rejection from friends and family, as well as the perceived social stigma and isolation related to the illness.

General Issues

 Assessment

A. Complete the basic triage assessment per protocol.
B. Perform a subjective assessment.
   1. Nonspecific symptoms:
      △ fever
      △ weakness
      △ malaise
      △ change in level of consciousness
      △ anorexia
      △ fatigue
      △ chills
   2. Specific symptoms:
      △ onset of symptoms
      △ exacerbating factors
      △ rate of symptom development
      △ response to any self-treatment
   3. Disease or drugs that would compromise patient's immune system:
      △ diabetes
      △ antibiotics
      △ cancer
      △ immunosuppressive drugs
      △ AIDS
      △ chemotherapy
      △ steroids
   4. High-risk patient populations:
      △ homeless
      △ incarcerated
      △ psychiatric
      △ sociopathic behavior
      △ alcohol or substance abuse
      △ age fragile (infant or elderly)
      △ day care centers
      △ prolonged immobility
      △ nursing homes

C. Peform an objective assessment.
  1. Neurologic findings:
     Δ confusion
     Δ apprehension
     Δ lethargy
     Δ agitation
  2. Vital signs:
     Δ fever
     Δ hypotension
     Δ orthostatic vitals signs
     Δ tachycardia
     Δ tachypnea
  3. Ears, nose, throat, and lymph nodes:
     Δ pain
     Δ swelling
     Δ discharge or exudate
     Δ lesions
     Δ erythema
  4. Chest:
     Δ lung sounds
     Δ heart sounds
     Δ productive cough
  5. Abdomen:
     Δ vomiting
     Δ diarrhea
     Δ bowel sounds
     Δ pain on palpation
  6. Genitals:
     Δ lesions
     Δ parasites
     Δ exudates
     Δ inflammation
  7. Skin or extremities:
     Δ cellulitis
     Δ warmth
     Δ swelling
     Δ purpura
     Δ tenderness
     Δ erythema
     Δ petechiae
     Δ joint pain
     Δ lesions
     Δ abscesses
     Δ nuchal rigidity
     Δ limited range of motion

Interventions

1. Will vary with each disease or infectious process
2. Consider isolation room based on patient history and assessment of current symptoms

Communicable Diseases

Communicable Diseases

Disease	Mode of Transmission	Incubation Period	Contagious Period
Acquired Immuno-deficiency Syndrome (AIDS) *Human Immunodeficiency Virus (HIV)*	Blood, breast milk, body tissues, fluids exchanged during sexual contact Other body fluids: saliva, urine, tears, bronchial secretions (especially if blood is present)	Variable incubation rates Virus exposure to seroconversion (HIV+): ~1–3 months HIV+ to AIDS from <1–10 years	Although unknown, it is believed to begin just after onset of HIV and extend throughout life
Botulism	Contaminated food products	Within 12–36 hours of consumption, up to several days	Not contagious from secondary person-to-person contact
Bronchiolitis	Respiratory	4–6 days	Onset of cough until 7 days
Chancroid	Direct sexual contact with open, or draining lesions	3–5 days up to 14 days	Until treated with antibiotic and lesions healed; usually about 1–2 weeks
Chicken pox (varicella) *Herpes zoster (shingles)*	Direct person-to-person contact Respiratory droplet Soiled dressings or articles	Commonly 14–16 days Can be 2–3 weeks	1–5 days before the onset of the rash, until all sores have crusted over, usually 10–21 days
Chlamydia	Sexual intercourse	Approximately 7–14 days	Unknown
"Cold," cough, croup	Respiratory	2–5 days	Onset of runny nose and/or cough until fever is gone
Conjunctivitis *Viral*	Direct or indirect contact	1–12 days	4–14 days after onset of symptoms (minimally contagious)
Bacterial	Respiratory Direct contact with eye drainage	24–72 hours	Until treated with antibiotics *continued*

Communicable Diseases (Continued)

Disease	Mode of Transmission	Incubation Period	Contagious Period
Fifth disease	Respiratory	Variable 4–20 days	7 days before rash develops, probably not communicable after rash starts
Giardia	Fecal contamination of food or water	3–25 days	Entire period of infection, often months
Gonorrhea	Sexual contact	2–7 days	Continues until treatment begins
Hand, foot and mouth disease (Coxsackie virus)	Direct contact with nasal or throat secretions, fecal Droplet	3–6 days	Onset of mouth ulcers until fever gone—perhaps as long as several weeks with fecal contamination
Hepatitis A	Fecal–oral route Food contamination	15–50 days	During last half of incubation period until after first week of jaundice
Hepatitis B	Blood, saliva, semen, vaginal fluid	45–180 days	Infective many weeks before onset of first symptom, until completion of acute clinical course of infection
Hepatitis C	Blood and plasma Percutaneous exposure	2 weeks–6 months	From 1+ weeks before onset of symptoms; may persist indefinitely
Herpes simplex *Type 1* *Type 2*	 Saliva Sexual contact (oral or genital)	 2–12 days 2–12 days	 From onset of sores to 7 weeks after recovery from stomatitis 7–12 days
Impetigo *Staph* *Strep*	 Hand–skin contact Respiratory droplet Direct contact	 4–10 days 1–3 days	 Until draining lesions heal Untreated: weeks–months Treated: 24 hours on antibiotics
Influenza	Airborne Direct contact	1–3 days	Children: 7 days Adults: 3–5 days
Kawasaki	Unknown Seasonal variation	Unknown	Unknown
Legionnaire pneumonia	Airborne	2–10 days	Person-to-person: none
Lice *Head/Body* *Pubic (crabs)*	 Direct contact, indirect contact with objects Sexual contact	 7–13 days Egg-to-egg cycle lasts 3 weeks	 Continuous if alive, until first treatment Live off host for 7–21 days Live off host for 2 days

Communicable Diseases (Continued)

Disease	Mode of Transmission	Incubation Period	Contagious Period
Lyme disease	Tickborne	3–32 days	Person-to-person: none
Measles (rubeola)	Airborne Direct contact with nasal secretions	7–18 days	Before the onset of symptoms to 4 days after the appearance of the rash
Meningitis *Bacterial: Meningococcal*	Direct contact: respiratory droplet from nose and mouth	2–10 days	Usually after 24 hours on antibiotic therapy
* Bacterial: Haemophilus*	Droplet from nose and mouth	2–4 days	Noncommunicable within 24–48 hours on antibiotic therapy
* Viral*	Varies with specific infectious agent		Variable, often approximately 7 days
Mononucleosis	Saliva	4–6 weeks	Prolonged, possibly a year
Pertussis	Direct contact Airborne droplet	6–20 days	Gradually decreases over 3 weeks
Pinworms	Direct transfer (anus to mouth) Indirect contact (infested bed, etc)	2–6 weeks	As long as females are alive Eggs survive for about 2 weeks
Rabies	Saliva Direct contact (bite, scratch) Indirect contact	3–8 weeks	3–7 days before the onset of symptoms
Ringworm *Tinea capitus (scalp)*	Direct skin-to-skin Indirect contact (cloth seats, combs, etc.)	10–14 days	Viable fungus may persist on contaminated articles for long periods of time
* Tinea corporis (body)*	Direct or indirect contact with infected people, articles, floors, benches, animals, shower stalls	4–10 days	While lesions are present and as long as viable fungus remains on articles
Rocky Mountain spotted fever	Tickborne	3–14 days	Noncommunicable person-to-person Tick remains infective for life, as long as 18 months
Roseola	Unknown Possibly saliva	10–15 days	Onset of fever until rash is gone
Rotavirus *Rotaviral enteritis*	Fecal–oral route Possible respiratory	24–72 hours	Average 4–6 days
Rubella	Direct contact nasal secretions Droplet	14–23 days	1 week before to at least 4 days after onset of rash

continued

Communicable Diseases (Continued)

Disease	Mode of Transmission	Incubation Period	Contagious Period
Salmonella	Ingestion of contaminated food	6–72 hours	Throughout the course of infection
Scabies	Direct skin-to-skin contact	2–6 weeks	Until mites and eggs are destroyed
Scarlet fever	Large respiratory droplet Direct contact	1–3 days	Untreated: 10–21 days Treated: 24 hours of antibiotic therapy
Shigella	Fecal–oral route Ingestion of contaminated food	12–96 hours	During acute infection until infectious agent no longer in feces (~4 weeks)
Sore throat			
Strep	Large respiratory droplet Direct contact	1–3 days	Untreated: 10–21 days Treated: after 24 hours of antibiotic therapy
Viral	Direct contact Inhalation of airborne droplet	1–5 days	Onset of sore throat until fever gone
Syphilis	Direct contact with moist lesions and body fluids	10 days–3 months	Untreated: variable and indefinite Treated: after 24–48 hours of antibiotic therapy
Tetanus	Spores enter open wound	3–21 days	Noncommunicable from person-to-person
Trichomoniasis	Sexual contact through vaginal or urethral secretions	4–24 days	Untreated: may be symptom-free carrier for years
Tuberculosis	Airborne droplet	4–12 weeks	Degree of communicability depends on many factors Treated: within a few weeks Children with TB usually not infectious

(NYSDOH, 1994; Benenson, 1995; Nettina, 1997)

Sexually Transmitted Diseases

Sexually Transmitted Diseases		
Disease	Clinical Presentation	Complications and Long-Term Risks
AIDS/HIV	May remain asymptomatic for many years Developing signs and symptoms include fatigue, fever, poor appetite, unexplained weight loss, generalized lymphadenopathy, persistent diarrhea, night sweats	Disease progression (from HIV to AIDS) is variable from a few months to 12 years Early intervention is essential in preserving and maintaining optimal health status
Chancroid	Painful genital ulceration(s) with tender inguinal adenopathy; ulcers may be necrotic or erosive	Chancroid has been associated with increased risk of acquiring HIV infection Should be tested for other infections that cause ulcers (e.g., syphilis)
Chlamydial cervicitis	Yellow mucopurulent cervical exudate May or may not be symptomatic Male sexual partner will likely have nongonococcal urethritis	Untreated, may develop endometritis, salpingitis, ectopic pregnancy, and/or subsequent infertility High prevalence of co-infection with gonococcal infection Infection during pregnancy may lead to premature rupture of the membranes; pneumonia or conjunctivitis in the infant
Enteric infections	Sexually transmissible enteric infections, particularly among homosexual males Abdominal pain, fever, diarrhea, vomiting	Occurs frequently with oral–genital and oral–anal contact Infections can be life-threatening if become systemic Organisms may be Shigella, hepatitis A, Giardia
Epididymitis	May or may not be transmitted sexually Can be asymptomatic Nonsexually transmitted, is associated with a urinary tract infection Unilateral testicular pain, swelling	Usually caused by gonorrhea or chlamydia May be caused by E. coli after anal intercourse Must rule out a testicular torsion before making the diagnosis of epididymitis
Genital warts	Soft, fleshy, painless growth(s) around the anus, penis, vulvovaginal area, cervix, urethra, or perineum	Caused by the human papillomavirus Must rule out other causes of lesion(s), such as syphilis, etc. Lesions may cause tissue destruction Cervical warts are associated with neoplasia

continued

Sexually Transmitted Diseases (Continued)

Disease	Clinical Presentation	Complications and Long-Term Risks
Gonorrhea	Males may have dysuria, urinary frequency, thin clear or yellow urethral discharge Females may have mucopurulent vaginal discharge, abnormal menses, dysuria, or may be asymptomatic	Untreated, risk of arthritis, dermatitis, bacteremia, meningitis, endocarditis At risk: males—epididymitis, infertility, urethral stricture, and sterility; females—pelvic inflammatory disease; newborns—ophthalmia neonatorum, pneumonia
Hepatitis B	Anorexia, malaise, nausea, vomiting, abdominal pain, jaundice, skin rash, arthralgias, arthritis	Chronic hepatitis, cirrhosis, liver cancer, liver failure, death Chronic carrier occurs in 6–10% of cases Infants born with hepatitis B are at high risk for developing chronic liver disease
Herpes Genitalis Herpes Simplex Type 2	Clustered vesicles that rupture, leaving painful, shallow genital ulcer(s) that eventually crust Initial outbreak last for 14–21 days; subsequent outbreaks are less severe and last 8–12 days	Other causes of genital ulcers (syphilis, chancroid, etc.) must be ruled out
Nongonococcal urethritis	Dysuria, urinary frequency, mucoid to purulent urethral discharge Some men may be asymptomatic Female sexual partners may have cervicitis or PID	Can be caused by chlamydia, mycoplasma, trichomonas, or herpes simplex Can cause urethral strictures, prostatitis, epididymitis
Pelvic Inflammatory Disease	Lower abdominal pain, fever, cervical motion tenderness, dyspareunia, purulent vaginal discharge, dysuria, increase abdominal pain while walking	Must rule out appendicitis or ectopic pregnancy Risk for pelvic abscess, future ectopic pregnancy, infertility, pelvic adhesions
Proctitis	Sexually transmitted gastrointestinal illnesses Proctitis occurs with anal intercourse, resulting in inflammation of the rectum with anorectal pain, tenesmus, and rectal discharge	May be caused by chlamydia, gonorrhea, herpes simplex, and syphilis Among patients co-infected with HIV, herpes proctitis may be severe
Proctocolitis	Sexually transmitted gastrointestinal illnesses Proctocolitis occurs with either anal intercourse or with oral–fecal contact, resulting in symptoms of proctitis as well as diarrhea, abdominal cramps, and inflammation of the colonic mucosa	May be caused by Campylobacter, Shigella, or chlamydia Other opportunistic infections may be involved among immunosuppressed HIV patients

Sexually Transmitted Diseases (Continued)

Disease	Clinical Presentation	Complications and Long-Term Risks
Pubic lice	Slight discomfort to intense itching May have pruritic, erythematous macules, papules, or secondary excoriation in the genital area	Sexual partners within the last month should be treated May develop lymphadenitis or a secondary bacterial infection of the skin or hair follicle
Scabies	The mite burrows under the skin of the fingers, penis, and wrists Scabies among adults may be sexually transmitted, while usually *not* sexually transmitted among children Itching (worse at night), papular eruptions, and excoriation of the skin	Sexual partners, household member, and close contacts within the past month should be examined and treated May develop a secondary infection, often with nephritogenic streptococci

Syphilis

Disease	Clinical Presentation	Complications and Long-Term Risks
Primary syphilis	Painless, indurated, ulcer (chancre) at site of infection approximately 10 days to 3 months after exposure	All genital ulcers should be suspected to be syphilitic Should be tested for HIV and retested again in 3 months
Secondary syphilis	Rash, mucocutaneous lesions, lymphadenopathy, condylomata lata Symptoms occur 4–6 weeks after exposure, and resolve spontaneously within weeks to 12 months	At-risk sexual partners are those within the past 3 months plus duration of symptoms for primary syphilis, and 6 months plus duration of symptoms for secondary syphilis
Latent syphilis	Seroreactive yet asymptomatic Can be clinically latent for a period of weeks to years Latency sometimes lasts lifetime	Should be clinically evaluated for tertiary disease (i.e., aortitis, neurosyphilis, etc.) At-risk sexual partners are those within the past year for early latent syphilis
Tertiary/Late syphilis	May have cardiac, neurologic, ophthalmic, auditory, or gummatous lesions	
Neurosyphilis	May see a variety of neurologic signs and symptoms, including ataxia, bladder problems, confusion, meningitis, uveitis May be asymptomatic	Diagnosis made based on a variety of tests, including reactive serologic test results, cerebrospinal fluid (CSF) protein or cell count abnormalities, positive VDRL on CSF
Congenital syphilis	Needs to be ruled out for infants born to mothers with untreated syphilis, mothers who received incomplete treatment, or insufficient follow-up of reported treated syphilis Serologic tests for mother and infant can be negative at delivery if mother was infected late in pregnancy	Syphilis frequently causes abortion, stillbirth, and complications of prematurity of infant Treated infants must be followed very closely and retested every 2–3 months Most infants are nonreactive by 6 months Infants with positive CSF should be retested every 6 months and be retreated if still abnormal at 2 years

continued

Sexually Transmitted Diseases (Continued)

Disease	Clinical Presentation	Complications and Long-Term Risks
Trichomoniasis vaginitis	Profuse, thin, foamy, greenish-yellow discharge with foul odor May be asymptomatic Male partners may have urethritis	Trichomoniasis often coexists with gonorrhea Perform a complete STD assessment if trichomoniasis is diagnosed

(USDHHS, 1990; Lippincott, 1991; NYSDOH, 1994; Benenson, 1995; Nettina, 1997)

■ UNIVERSAL PRECAUTIONS

The triage nurse must practice according to the guidelines of universal precautions for each and every patient who enters the department for care. It is important to remember each patient is potentially the carrier of a contagious disease. The Occupational Safety and Health Administration (OSHA) maintains strict standards that apply to everyone who is at risk of coming into contact with blood or body fluids during the performance of routine job duties. It is up to the individual employee and each facility to know and adhere to the current standards of universal precautions.

In addition to blood, other potentially infectious materials include:

- semen
- vaginal secretions
- cerebrospinal fluid
- synovial fluid
- any body fluid visibly contaminated with blood
- any unidentifiable body fluids
- peritoneal fluid
- amniotic fluid
- saliva

The goal of universal precautions is to minimize or eliminate the significant health risk posed by occupational exposure to blood and other potentially infectious materials that may contain blood-borne pathogens. Among the diseases that healthcare workers are at risk of contracting are hepatitis B, human immunodeficiency virus (HIV), hepatitis C, syphilis, and other contagious blood-borne diseases.

Gloves, goggles, and masks should routinely be stocked in the triage room and utilized by the triage nurse. Good handwashing or the use of an approved hand disinfectant is essential between patients. Hands should always be washed immediately on the removal of gloves.

Red bag or biohazard trash receptacles should be available for the disposal of contaminated products and used for all potentially contaminated trash.

It is important for the triage nurse to include the patient when utilizing universal precautions and to educate the patient about the need for such special care. Patients may be anxious regarding the use of protective wear, and simple patient education can help reduce their anxiety. The triage nurse should also take a proactive role in teaching young children who may be curious and attracted to the brightly colored biohazard receptacle, and keep them from playing with these trash cans.

Isolation

Any patient who presents with a potentially contagious skin rash must be escorted directly from the triage room into the department's isolation room. This room may also be utilized for enteric precautions. The patient should be taught the importance of this isolation and kept from walking through the main ED whenever possible.

Any patient who presents with a potentially contagious respiratory condition should be considered for placement in the negative pressure room (if your department has one). If the patient's condition is of high acuity, the triage nurse should decide which bed in the ED will best suit the patient's needs and maintain respiratory isolation within that examination room. The patient should wear a mask when being transported through the department or the facility hallways.

A patient presenting with chicken pox must be placed in the isolation room and be isolated for both respiratory and contact isolation.

After the discharge of a patient with a contagious illness, the room must be thoroughly decontaminated per hospital policy.

MENTAL HEALTH

Δ A mental health emergency is any alteration in thought process, feelings, or actions for which immediate therapeutic interventions are indicated.

Δ It is essential to develop rapport quickly with the patient, as this has a great impact on the nurse's ability to accurately complete the triage assessment of him or her.

ALERT

Δ The nature and degree of the mental health crisis that brings a person to the ED is defined primarily by the person experiencing it.

Δ Exception: Psychotic patients who are out of touch with reality fail to realize they are in any sort of difficulty.

Δ What may seem insignificant to the health care team may be perceived by the patient as an overwhelming event, feeling, or thought.

Δ Patients may feel vulnerable, frightened, and out of control. The triage nurse *must* convey empathy, respect, and understanding to the patient.

Δ A prompt assessment is essential to determine the risk patients pose to themselves or others.

General Issues

Assessment

A. Obtain and record complete triage assessment:
   1. Perform a basic triage assessment per protocol.
   2. Obtain a history of chief complaint.
      Δ Current symptoms, including:
         • nature
         • onset
         • duration
      Δ In the presence of delusions or hallucinations, consider asking:
         • "Are you hearing voices?"
         • "What are the voices telling you?"
         • "Do you want to hurt yourself? Someone else?"
      Δ Recent changes:
         • life stressors
         • medication
         • sexual interest
         • appetite
         • sleep pattern
         • digestive functions
         • level of functioning:
            * socially
            * physically

        * occupationally

        * mentally

3. Obtain a past history.
   - Δ Medical
     - head trauma
     - Alzheimer's
     - brain tumor
     - infections
     - hypoxia
     - renal failure
     - seizure disorder
     - multiple sclerosis
     - endocrine dysfunctions
     - metabolic abnormalities
     - alcohol intoxication or withdrawal
     - metabolic abnormalities
     - drug ingestion (PCP, LSD, cocaine, etc.)
     - liver failure
     - nutritional deficiencies
     - AIDS-related dementia
   - Δ Psychiatric
     - anxiety
     - somatoform disorders
     - schizophrenia
     - eating disorders
     - personality disorders (obsessive/compulsive, borderline, etc.)
     - depression
     - bipolar (manic depression)
     - suicidal or homicidal behavior
     - sexual and gender identity disorders
   - Δ Familial
     - substance abuse
     - domestic violence
     - mental illness among family members
     - income level
     - living arrangements

4. Perform a physical assessment.
   - Δ Assess for:
     - diaphoresis
     - agitation
     - cool, clammy skin
     - tachycardia
     - thought process
     - anxiety
     - pallor

- flushing
- dystonic movements
- speech irregularities
- respiratory distress or tachypnea
- motor restlessness or pacing

5. Perform a mental status examination.
   - Δ Assess for obvious changes in behavior, speech, thought process.
   - Δ Refer to "Pearls of Triage Wisdom: Mental Health" (later in this book) for a complete description of how to perform a mental status exam.
6. Consider the patient's age.
   - Δ Pediatric or adolescent
     - Age-appropriate behaviors vary.
     - Differentiation between abnormal behavior or normal adjustment behavior is difficult.
     - Assess for:
       - * extreme sadness
       - * overreacts frequently
       - * extremely fearful
       - * poor concentration
       - * chemical dependency
       - * drop in school grades
       - * defiance of rules
       - * switching friends
       - * change in behavior
       - * inflicts harm on others
       - * persistent nightmares
       - * anorexia or bulimia
       - * breaks the law
       - * hopelessness
       - * constant or extreme anger
       - * cries easily for "no reason"
       - * desires to be alone constantly
       - * possibility of abuse or assault
       - * secrecy or isolation
       - * emotional highs and lows
       - * withdrawal from family and friends
       - * drop in work or sport performance
       - * focused on topics such as death
       - * abuses laxatives
       - * destroys property
       - * performs life-threatening acts
   - Δ Elderly
     - Assess for:
       - * chemical dependency
       - * cognitive impairment
       - * organic manifestations

* withdrawal or isolation
* social stressors
* personal loss
* thorough review of medications (prescriptions, OTC, natural or home remedies)

Interventions

1. Protect safety of patient, staff, and visitors. Involve security as needed or indicated per hospital protocol.
2. Listen to patient and acknowledge statements.
3. Focus on the patient's safety and needs; work to develop rapport.
4. Avoid condescending speech, threatening movements, or any staff behavior that would further aggravate the patient.
5. Remove high-risk patients to a quiet yet closely monitored setting as soon as possible:
   Δ patients at risk of harming self or others
   Δ agitated patients
   Δ survivors of domestic violence
   Δ confused patients

Alcohol Abuse, Alcoholism, and Alcohol Withdrawal

Δ It is estimated that 18 million people abuse alcohol.
Δ Alcohol is involved in:
- 86% of homicides
- 65% of suicide completions
- 60% of sexual offenses
- 60% of boating fatalities
- 57% of men involved in marital violence
- 42% of violent crime
- 40% of all traffic fatalities
- 27% of women involved in marital violence (NIAAA, 1994; NIAAA, 1997; Wolbert, 1997; Varcarcolis, 1998)

The nurse should always stay alert for signs of alcohol use or abuse and carefully utilize any information gathered when assigning a triage acuity and formulating a plan of care for the patient.

Assessment

A. Perform a general mental health assessment per protocol.
   1. Associated information:
      Δ description of current drinking episode
      Δ pattern of drinking behavior

Δ length of time since last drink

Δ presence of poly-substance abuse

2. Physical findings or medical history of:

Δ poor dentition

Δ hoarseness

Δ esophageal varices

Δ arrhythmias

Δ ascites

Δ liver enlargement

Δ myopathy

Δ skin lesions

Δ gout

Δ hypoglycemia

Δ delirium tremens

Δ seizures

Δ hepatic disease

Δ ulcers/gastritis

Δ frequent respiratory infections

Δ cardiomyopathy

Δ memory deficits

Δ sleep disturbances

Δ cerebellar degeneration

Δ "blackouts"

Δ hallucinations (usually visual or tactile)

3. Signs of alcohol intoxication:

Δ unsteady gait

Δ incoordination

Δ nystagmus

Δ belligerence

Δ odor of alcohol

Δ mood lability

Δ impaired judgement

Δ vomiting

Δ palpitations

Δ stupor

Δ slurred speech

Δ confusion

Δ impaired attention

Δ loss of inhibition

Δ altered level of perception

Δ memory loss

Δ hypertension

Δ cardiac arrhythmias

Δ coma

4. Signs of alcohol withdrawal:
   May *begin* 6–8 hours after cessation or reduction of the alcohol intake, and symptoms will *peak* in approximately 24–48 hours.
   Δ Stage 1
   - anxiety
   - tachycardia
   - nausea/vomiting
   - headache
   - insomnia
   - dehydration
   - tremors
   - diaphoresis
   - nightmares
   - anorexia
   - hypertension
   - hypovolemia
   - irritability
   - depression
   - positive orthostatic vital signs
   - jerky muscle movements
   - hyperthermia
   Δ Stage 2
   - hallucinations (tactile, visual, auditory)
   - intensification of stage 1 symptoms
   Δ Stage 3
   - paranoia
   - delirium
   - disorientation
   - delusions
   - amnesia
   - intensification of stage 1 and 2 symptoms
   Δ Stage 4
   - seizures

ALERT Appropriate identification and treatment before the development of stages 1 and 2 *prevent* stages 3 and 4.

Facts:

Δ Mortality rate for delerium tremens (DT) is 20%.

Δ DTs are preventable with sedatives.

Δ It is difficult to predict which patients will develop a major withdrawal reaction; therefore, it is reasonable to sedate all patients who are recently abstinent from alcohol.

Δ It is difficult to control a severe withdrawal reaction once it begins; therefore, aggressive therapy of all early abstinence patients is important.

Δ Large doses of sedatives may be required to prevent severe withdrawal reaction and DTs.

   B. If suspicion of alcoholism exists, perform a more specific substance abuse assessment.

      1. History of substances:

         Δ age substance first used

         Δ frequency, amount, and duration of use

         Δ date or time of last use for each of the following:

- alcohol
- cocaine/crack
- cannabis
- depressants
- heroin
- inhalants
- hallucinogens
- stimulants
- other (including prescribed medications)

      2. History of:

         Δ withdrawal

         Δ tolerance

         Δ previous treatment programs (including when and where)

- inpatient
- outpatient
- self-help

         Δ success with previous programs

         Δ family history of substance abuse

      3. CAGE questions:

         Δ **C** Have you ever attempted to *cut down* on your use?

         Δ **A** Have you ever been *annoyed* when others mention your use?

         Δ **G** Have you ever felt *guilty* about your use?

         Δ **E** Have you ever needed an *"eye opener"?*

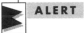 **ALERT**   Two or three "yes" answers to these questions strongly suggest chemical dependence.

Interventions

 ALERT   Withdrawal from alcohol is a potentially lethal process.

1. Complete primary and secondary survey with interventions as indicated.
2. Assess for suicidal behavior.
3. Check blood pressure, pulse, and temperature readings hourly for the first 8–12 hours after admission.
   Δ Vital signs should be assessed at least every 4 hours for the first 48 hours after admission (Varcarolis, 1998).
   Δ The pulse is a good indicator of progression into and through withdrawal.
   Δ Elevated pulse may indicate pending alcohol withdrawal delirium.
4. Obtain intravenous access for rehydration.
   Δ Because of hypoglycemia, hypokalemia, hypomagnesemia, and thiamine deficiency that are common to the alcoholic person, replacements must be given at the time of intravenous (IV) initiation.

 ALERT   Thiamine must be replaced prior to the administration of glucose to prevent the development of Wernicke-Korsakoff syndrome (Kitt et al., 1995).

5. Administer medication as patient progresses through withdrawal. (Phenobarbital and lorazepam are most commonly used.)

Bipolar Disorder (Manic/Depression)

Δ Bipolar disorder is a mood disorder characterized by alternating manic and depressive episodes.
Δ Manic episodes include extremely labile excitement, hyperactivity, and euphoria.
Δ Depressive episodes include extreme sadness, slowed thought process, and marked fatigue.
Δ The patient may have long periods of normal and stable moods between elevated and depressed moods.

 ALERT   Patient is a threat to himself and others until *mania* is controlled or severe *depression* is relieved.

Assessment

A. Perform a general mental health assessment per protocol.
  1. Associated information:
     Δ complete medical history and triage assessment
     Δ organic causes of depression
     Δ electroconvulsive therapy that may precipitate a manic episode
     Δ medication that may cause episodes of mania:
       • antidepressants
       • amphetamines
       • steroids
     Δ medications that may cause depression:
       • antihypertensives
       • oral contraceptives
       • steroids
       • narcotics
       • antiparkinsonian drugs
       • amphetamines
       • barbiturates
     Δ family history of bipolar illness
     Δ previous episodes of manic/depression
  2. Associated signs and symptoms of mania:
     Δ three most common symptoms of mania include:
       • elated mood
       • increased activity
       • reduced sleep
     Δ other signs and symptoms include:
       • flight of ideas
       • grandiosity
       • inflated self-esteem
       • impaired mentation
       • flamboyant actions
       • disorganized behavior
       • hyperactivity
       • auditory hallucinations
       • psychosis
       • increased sexual energy
       • impairment of rational thought
       • poor social judgment
       • hostile or paranoid behavior when stressed
       • impulsive behavior
       • sleep impairment
       • rapid or pressured speech
       • excessive spending
       • boundless enthusiasm
  3. Associated signs and symptoms of depression (see Mental Health/Depression).

Interventions

1. Complete primary and secondary survey with interventions as indicated.
2. Provide for patient safety.
   Δ security officers
   Δ possibility of chemical and/or physical restraints
3. Remain emotionally separated from patient's behavior.
   Δ Although the patient may present as humorous, joking, and full of energy, the nurse must remain professional at all times.
   Δ Move the patient from a stimulating environment into a quiet one.
   Δ Set limits and enforce them.
   - The manic patient may attempt to control decisions and boundaries.
   - Staff must follow established policies and plans of care for this patient.

Depression

Δ Depression is an affective disorder that affects most people at some point in their life.
Δ It causes intense emotional pain and suffering.
Δ Depression may potentially be linked to suicide.
Δ It can be difficult to diagnose, as it is easily masked by somatic symptoms and has a variety of manifestations, intensities, and etiologies.
Δ Depression affects at least 10 million Americans.
Δ It is difficult to diagnose in adolescence because:
- teens may be ambivalent about sharing feelings with adults
- symptoms may be dismissed as "a stage they're going through"
- acting out behavior may mask depression

Assessment

A. Perform a general mental health assessment per protocol.
1. Associated information:
   Δ complete medical history and triage assessment
   Δ rule out:
   - possibility of organic cause of depression
   - increased use of alcohol, prescriptions, or OTC medications
   - use of medications that may cause depression, such as:
     * antihypertensives
     * oral contraceptives
     * steroids
     * narcotics
     * antiparkinsonian drugs
     * amphetamines
     * barbiturates
     * inhalants

Δ situational crisis
- loss of significant other
- sudden health changes
- separation from spiritual source or normal support system
- childbirth
- change in occupational status

2. Associated signs and symptoms:
   Δ extreme fatigue
   Δ anhedonia
   Δ changes in appetite
   Δ overwhelming sense of hopelessness and helplessness
   Δ persistent irritability
   Δ sense of guilt or worthlessness
   Δ somatic complaints with no organic cause
   Δ forgetfulness
   Δ impairment of sleep pattern
   - difficulty falling asleep
   - difficulty staying asleep
   - excessive sleep
   Δ psychomotor agitation
   - depressed mood
   - crying
   Δ psychomotor retardation
   - slowed metabolism
   - monotone voice
   - constipation
   - slowed speech process
   - minimal body movement
   - slowed thought process
   Δ thoughts of death or suicide

 ALERT Thoughts of suicide should *always* be taken seriously. Complete a suicide risk assessment.

3. Age-related considerations:
   Δ Pediatric patients may present with:
   - hyperactivity
   - enuresis
   - regression
   - aggression
   - sadness
   - sleeping problems
   - irritability

- anxiety
- suicidal ideation
- misbehavior
- restlessness
- change in appetite

△ Adolescents may present with:
- acting out behaviors
- delinquency
- detached from others
- anger or hostility
- hopelessness
- alcohol and drug abuse
- aggression
- suicidal ideation
- verbal sarcasm
- traumatic injuries
- school issues
- disillusionment
- loneliness
- sexual promiscuity
- overeating or anorexia
- conduct disorders
- running away from home
- preoccupation with death

 ALERT Persistent or sudden signs of change can be key in identification of depression in adolescence.

△ Elderly may present with:
- apathy
- loss of appetite
- insomnia
- weight loss
- mood swings
- easy agitation
- pessimism
- extreme fatigue
- low self-esteem
- suicidal thoughts
- profound memory impairment
- very unsociable behavior
- change in sleep patterns
- decreased sexual activity

- heightened concerns for bodily functions
- increased anxiety and fear for no reason
- feelings of insignificance
- inability to concentrate
- poor personal hygiene
- delusions of persecution or somatic theme

 ALERT A depressed elderly person may appear to have dementia, not depression. Assess *carefully!*

 Interventions

1. Complete primary and secondary survey with interventions as indicated.
2. Assess for patient safety and assign patient to treatment area as necessary.
3. Arrange for 1:1 observation if patient at risk for suicide.
4. Form a therapeutic relationship with the patient, which includes excellent communication skills, empathy, trust, and compassion.
5. Avoid labeling an elderly patient as "demented" until a complete mental health assessment has been performed.
6. If you suspect that a depressed patient may be suicidal, ask:
   Δ "Sometimes when people feel this depressed/hopeless/sad, they have thoughts of hurting or killing themselves. Have you ever had thoughts like these?"
   Δ If the patient answers "yes," then assess the following:
   - Does the person have a plan?
   - Assess lethality of plan (handful of aspirin versus a gun)
   - Does person have the means to carry out the plan?
   - Does he or she have access to a gun, poison, car, and so on?
   - Has person ever attempted suicide before?

Drugs of Abuse

Drug Type/Drug Name	Street Name	Method Used	Physical Effects	Mental Effects
Alcohol				
CNS depressant (>10 million alcoholics in the United States	Booze Hooch Juice Brew	Swallowed in liquid form	Blurs vision, slurs speech, alters coordination, heart and liver damage, addiction, gastric and esophageal ulcers, brain damage, blackouts, hypoglycemia, anemia, Wernicke-Korsakoff syndrome, oral cancer, fetal alcohol syndrome, death from overdose	Scrambles thought process, impairs judgment, memory loss, alters perception, delirium, apathy
Cocaine				
CNS stimulant	Coke C-dust Snow Toot White lady Blow Rock(s) Crack Flake Big "C" Happy dust Bernice Horse Fluff Caine Coconut Icing Mojo Zip	Smoked/free basing, inhaled/snorted injected, swallowed in powder, pill or rock form	Rapidly metabolized, producing a brief high of <30 minutes; chronic use can result in cocaine psychosis, a condition similar to paranoid schizophrenia, intense psychological dependence, dilated pupils, profuse sweating, runny nose, dry mouth, tachycardia, hypertension, insomnia, anorexia, indifference to pain, destruction of nasal septum, heart and lung damage, death from overdose	Euphoria, illusive mental or physical power, extreme mood swings, restlessness, hallucinations, paranoia, psychosis, severe depression, anxiety, formication
CNS depressants				
Barbiturates				
phenobarbital: Luminal amobarbital: Amytal secobarbital: Seconal pentobarbital: Nembutal	Reds Barbs Yellow Jackets Red Devils	IV injection, suppository, swallowed in pill form	Drowsiness, slurred speech, skeletal muscle relaxation, poor muscle control, incoordination, nausea, slowed reaction time, involuntary eye movements, hypotension, bradycardia,	Confusion, impaired judgment, impaired performance, anxiety and tension followed by a sense of calm, mood swings, forgetfulness

continued

Drug Type/Drug Name	Street Name	Method Used	Physical Effects	Mental Effects
Barbiturates (continued,) sodium pentothal	Blue Devils Yellow Submarine Blues and Reds Idiot pills Sleepers Stumblers Downers		bradypnea, constricted pupils, clammy skin, loss of appetite; penetrates the placental wall; addiction is passed to the baby, withdrawal is prolonged and severe—symptoms range from temporary psychosis to cardiac arrest; cellulitis at injection site; chronic use results in extreme psychological and physical addiction; death from overdose	
Nonbarbiturate Methaqualone Quaalude Soper	Downers Ludes Soapers Wallbangers Lemons Lovers Quack 714s 300s	Swallowed in pill form	Same as barbiturates, physically and psychologically addictive, withdrawal is *very* difficult, severe interaction with alcohol, death from overdose	Same as barbiturates
Tranquilizers, Benzodiazepines (Reduces tension and anxiety without sedating) diazepam: Valium chlordiazepoxide: Librium lorazepam: Ativan oxazepam: Serax alprazolam: Xanax	Downers	Injected, swallowed in pill form	Decreased reflex action, vision changes, muscle relaxation, hypotension, bradycardia, drowsiness, slurred speech, blurred vision; prolonged use causes severe physical and psychological addition	Alteration in spatial judgment and sense of time, sense of calm, impaired judgment, confusion, depression, hallucinations
Hallucinogens (Drugs that alter perceptions of reality) PCP	Angel dust Killer Black whack Supergrass Peace pill Sherms	Swallowed in pill form, sprayed on a cigarette and smoked	Drooling, nystagmus, restlessness, incoordination, rigid muscles, tachycardia, hypertension, superhuman strength, dulled sensations to touch and pain, impaired speech; death is common, but from accidents, not	Disorientation, amnesia, anxiety, depression, confusion, agitation, violent, hostile, suicidal, extreme personality changes

Drug	Street Names	Route	Effects	
	Superweed, DOA, CJ, Goon dust, Dust joint, Live one, Mad dog, T-buzz, Wobble weed, Zombie		from overdose; extremely dangerous drug as it is a narcotic, stimulant, depressant, and hallucinogen; a "trip" is a cycle of stimulation, depression, hallucination, and then repeats itself, lasting 2–14 hours	

Hallucinogens (*Drugs that alter perceptions of reality*)

Drug	Street Names	Route	Physical Effects	Psychological Effects
LSD	Acid, Blue Heaven, Instant Zen, Purple Hearts, Pure Love, Sugar Cubes, Tail lights	Swallowed in liquid form, dropped on sugar cube, sprayed on paper tablet	Nausea, tachycardia, tachypnea, hyperthermia, hypertension, dilated pupils, diaphoresis, palpitations, incoordination; trips last 4–14 hours; heightens all five senses	Altered reality perception, psychotic disturbances, paranoia, synesthesia, hallucinations, mood swings, terrifying flashbacks
Mescaline, Psilocybin	Mesc, Moon, Peyote, Buttons	Swallowed in natural form	Same as LSD	Same as LSD

Inhalants

Drug	Street Names	Route	Physical Effects	Psychological Effects
Gasoline, Airplane glue, Paint thinner, Dry cleaner fluid, Nitrous oxide	Laughing gas, Whippets, Buzz Bomb, Nitro	Inhaled or sniffed using paper or plastic bag or rag; Inhaled or sniffed by mask or balloons	Incoordination, impaired vision, neuropathy, muscle weakness, anemia, vertigo, headache, weight loss, brain, liver, and bone marrow damage, death by anoxia	Memory and thought impairment, abusive behavior, violent
Amyl nitrite, Butyl nitrite	Poppers, Snappers, Pearls, Aimies, Bolt, Climax, Thrust	Inhaled or sniffed from gauze or ampules		

continued

Drugs of Abuse (Continued)

Drug Type/Drug Name		Street Name	Method Used	Physical Effects	Mental Effects
Marijuana/Hashish (a CNS depressant)		Joint Grass Hash Pot "J" Maryjane Reefer Colombian Locoweed Love weed	Smoked, swallowed in solid form	Interferes with psychological maturation; psychological dependence	Sensory distortion, decrease in motivation, forgetfulness, confusion, anxiety, paranoia
Narcotics (Natural or synthetic drugs that contain or resemble opium; CNS depressants)	Dilaudid Percodan Demerol Methadone	Dillys Cowboys Perks Pink spoons Peth Dollies Amidone Fizzies	Swallowed in pill or liquid form, injected	Drowsiness, lethargy, hypotension, bradycardia, muscle weakness, death from overdose	Forgetfulness, sedation, sense of peace
	Codeine	Schoolboy Cody Threes Fours	Swallowed in pill or liquid form		
	Morphine	Mojo Morphy Mud Dreamer Miss Emma	Smoked, IV injection	Tolerance occurs quickly; addiction occurs in as little as 1–3 weeks; withdrawal is painful with intense cramps, cold sweats, delirium, pain, fever, headaches and seizures lasting ~4 days	Produces an intense orgasmic rush followed by euphoria, peace, and a comforting warmth, confusion, forgetfulness, stupor
	Heroin	Horse Junk Dope Blanco Black pearl Bonita			

Drug	Form	Physical Effects	General Effects

Stimulants
(cause CNS stimulation)
 	
Amphetamines
Benzadrine
Biphetamine
 	
Dextroamphetamine
Dexedrine
Synatan
Appetral
Methamphetamine
Methedrine
Desoxyn
Ambar
	Pill form,
	injected,
	snorted
	
	Hi Speed
	Lip poppers
	Speckled
	  birds
	Dexies
	Brownies
	Brown and
	  clears
	Speed
	Meth
	Crystal
	Crank
	Crypto
	Ice
	Yellow bam
		Body enters a state of stress; anorexia, tachycardia, palpitations, hypertension, inability to sleep, nasal and bronchial passages enlarge, restriction of cerebral blood flow, dilated pupils, sweating, restlessness, muscle tremors, rapid and garbled speech, excessive activity, brain damage, seizures, CVA, coma, death from overdose; drug effects last 4–14 hours, "speeding" occurs with injection, causing user to go ~5 days without sleep; causes birth defects, extreme physical and psychological addiction	Extreme exhilaration and stimulation, inflated confidence, irritability, volatile, aggressive, nervousness, mood swings, hallucinations, paranoia, formication, psychosis, hypomania

Herbal stimulants Ephedrine Ultimate Xphoria Herbal Ecstasy Legal Weed Buzz Tablets Cloud 9 Black Lemonade Brainalizer Fungalore Herbal XTC Planet X The Drink X Tablets Brain Wash Buzz Tablets Fukola Cola Love Potion #69 Naturally High Rave Energy	Pill, powder, liquid	Same as above; often marketed as safe and legal alternatives to street drugs; package labels claim or imply similar high as street drugs, such as euphoria, natural high, heightened sexual sensation, higher energy level; easily obtainable over the Internet, through magazines, and at stores such as convenience markets, health food stores, and "head shops"	Same as above

Obsessive/Compulsive Disorder (OCD)

Δ An *obsession* is a persistent, intrusive, or unwanted thought or image that cannot be eliminated by reason or logic.

Δ *Compulsions* are repetitive behaviors performed to reduce or prevent the intense anxiety associated with the obsessive thought.

Δ Mild obsessive/compulsive symptoms are similar to someone who "worries too much." These obsessions are often socially acceptable (e.g., being on time) and only mildly annoying.

Δ More serious obsessive/compulsive behaviors involve sexuality, violence, germs, illness, or death. Those with a profound obsessive/compulsive disorder experience interpersonal, social, and economic dysfunction.

Δ Depression is suffered by 50% of patients with OCD (Varcarolis, 1994).

Assessment

A. Perform a general mental health assessment per protocol.
  1. Associated information:
     Δ may be ultimate perfectionist
     Δ great fear of making a mistake or being wrong
     Δ high emotional need to be in control
  2. Associated signs and symptoms:
     Δ skin or dental trauma from repeated cleansing
     Δ lack of appropriate coping skills
     Δ moderate to severe anxiety
     Δ impaired interpersonal relationships
     Δ fear
     Δ hypochondriacal behavior
     Δ pathological sense of guilt
     Δ chemical dependency
  3. Common obsessive thoughts:
     Δ checking and double-checking
     Δ sexual imagery or ideation
     Δ violent thought or acts against self or others
     Δ intense fear of germs or dirt
     Δ fear of illness or death
  4. Common compulsive behaviors:
     Δ counting (stairs, doors, cups, etc.)
     Δ touching (doorknobs, religious objects, etc.)
     Δ washing (hands, surfaces, objects, etc.)
     Δ avoiding (touching, people, groups, etc.)
     Δ doing/undoing (gets up from a chair and sits down again repeatedly)
     Δ symmetry (placing objects in perfect alignment, mandatory sequence, etc.)

Interventions

1. Complete primary and secondary survey with intervention as indicated.
2. Assess for patient safety and assign patient to treatment area as necessary.
3. Allow the patient time to complete the compulsive tasks.
4. Develop rapport with the patient to help decrease his or her heightened anxiety level.
5. Emphasize the patient's strengths.

Panic Attack/Disorder

Δ A spontaneous yet terrorizing emotional event experienced by a patient.
Δ This emotionally paralyzing event lasts for 3–10 minutes, and may include:
- suspension of normal function
- dramatically narrowed perceptual field
- misinterpretation of reality
- overwhelming fear or dread
- physical symptoms such as chest pain, shortness of breath, and so on.

Δ Depression may be suffered by 50–65% of the patients experiencing panic attacks (DSM-IV, 1994).

Assessment

A. Perform a general mental health assessment per protocol.
　1. Associated information:
　　Δ complete medical history and triage assessment
　　Δ situation that may precipitate a panic attack:
　　　- hypoglycemia
　　　- caffeine use
　　　- withdrawal from alcohol or tranquilizers
　　　- stressful event
　　　- sudden loss or life change
　2. Associated signs and symptoms:
　　Δ tachycardia
　　Δ dyspnea
　　Δ chest pain
　　Δ dizziness
　　Δ numbness, hands or feet
　　Δ delusions
　　Δ tremors
　　Δ overwhelming fear of losing control, going crazy, or dying
　　Δ palpitations
　　Δ tachypnea
　　Δ cool, clammy skin
　　Δ syncope

Δ hot or cold flashes
Δ hallucinations
Δ loss of reality orientation

Interventions

1. Complete primary and secondary survey with interventions as indicated.
2. Rule out physical cause for symptoms.
3. Provide for patient safety.
4. Stay with patient while offering reassurance.
5. Remove patient from stimulating environment.

Schizophrenia

Δ A pathological process resulting in psychotic behavior (acute or chronic)
Δ A severe disturbance in thought process, affect, behavior, and perception
Δ Impairment of reality orientation
Δ Severe withdrawal from reality and seclusion into a private world of his or her own
Δ Symptoms usually manifest during adolescence or early adulthood
Δ Slow onset, from 1 month to 2 years before the first psychotic break; may see gradual deterioration from previous level of functioning

Assessment

A. Perform a general mental health assessment per protocol.
 1. Associated information:
  Δ complete medical history and triage assessment
  Δ affect:
   • blunted
   • inappropriate
   • flat
   • bizarre
  Δ behavioral effects:
   • acting-out behavior
   • impulsiveness
   • catatonia
   • psychomotor retardation
   • psychomotor agitation
   • bizarre behaviors (i.e., eccentric dress)
  Δ perceptual effects:
   • illusions
   • derealization

- hallucinations
- autism
- depersonalization
- thinking not bound to reality

Δ impaired thought process
- delusions
- incoherence
- paranoia
- neologisms
- looseness of association
- confused
- illogical thought
- illogical speech (i.e., word salad)

Δ functional psychosis includes:
- schizophrenia
- mania
- psychotic depression
- brief reactive psychosis

Δ organic psychoses includes:
- dementia
- delirium
- toxic drug psychosis

2. Associated signs and symptoms:
Δ anhedonia
Δ acute or chronic anxiety
Δ loss of concentration
Δ loneliness
Δ lack of self-respect
Δ feelings of rejection
Δ compulsions and/or obsessions
Δ apathy
Δ uncommunicative speech
Δ delusions and/or hallucinations
Δ bizarre behavior
Δ poor social functioning
Δ vague or unrealistic future plans
Δ depression
Δ phobias
Δ inability to cope with environment
Δ hopelessness
Δ growing inability to trust others
Δ increasing sense of isolation
Δ appearance of talking to himself or herself
Δ agitation
Δ looseness of association

Interventions

1. Complete primary and secondary survey with interventions as indicated.
2. Assess for safety of patient, staff, and surrounding environment (i.e., waiting room).
3. Arrange for 1:1 observation if patient is a risk to him- or herself or others.
   Δ Notify security per facility policy.
4. Use therapeutic communication at all times.
   Δ Avoid threatening questions, including those that ask "why."
   Δ Avoid making assumptions when reflecting back a patient's statement.
   Δ Restate the person's statement to expand on their thought.
5. If patient is hearing voices, ask the patient what the voices are saying. Present the patient with reality by saying:
   Δ "I can see you are really frightened, but I don't hear any voices."
   Δ "Tell me, what do you hear them saying?"

Suicidal Behavior

Δ Suicide is the ninth leading cause of death in the United States.
  • It is the third leading cause of death among young people.
  • The highest rate of suicide is for persons over the age of 65.
  • Every 16.8 minutes someone kills him- or herself.
Δ It is estimated that:
  • 775,000 American attempt suicide each year.
  • There is a 0.5–1% completion (death) rate among the nation's young.
  • There is a 25% completion rate among the nation's elderly.
  • There are 10 to 25 attempts for every one suicide completion.
  • Each suicide intimately affects at least six other people.
Δ 75% of people who commit suicide send signals to those around them within 1 to 4 months prior to their death.
Δ Most people who attempt suicide are ambivalent about dying (Kitt, 1995; Anderson, 1997; Varcarolis, 1998).

ALERT   Nurses **must** take every suicidal gesture *seriously.*

Assessment

A. Perform a general mental health assessment per protocol.
  1. Associated information:
     Δ complete medical history and triage assessment
     Δ determine precipitating factors or events ("what makes today different?")
     Δ history of:
       • substance abuse
       • head trauma
       • psychosis
       • violent behavior
       • schizophrenia
       • aggression
       • borderline personality
       • organic diseases (e.g., temporal lobe epilepsy)
       • depression
       • abuse or assault
       • suicidal ideation
       • previous suicide attempts
       • impulsivity
       • family history of suicide
       • chronic or disabling disease
  2. Associated signs, symptoms, signals surrounding suicidal behavior:
     Δ giving possessions away
     Δ unusual peace or serenity
     Δ ambivalence
     Δ unnecessary risk taking
     Δ trouble sleeping
     Δ talk about death
     Δ refusal of basic essentials (food, meds, etc.)
     Δ lack of interest in personal hygiene
     Δ behavioral changes
     Δ increased used of drugs or alcohol
  3. Age-specific considerations:
     Δ Pediatric patients:
       • unusual changes in behavior
         * shy child becomes a thrill seeker
         * outgoing child becomes withdrawn and disinterested
       • giving possessions away
       • sadness, despair, depression
       • irritable or depressed moods
       • victim of sexual, physical, or emotional abuse
       • writes or draws pictures about death

△ Adolescents:
- depression
- impulsive behavior
- trouble sleeping
- hopelessness
- rebellious behavior
- preoccupation with death
- suddenly seems happy after being sad for a long time
- conduct disorders
- social withdrawal from friends
- appetite disturbances
- helplessness
- chemical dependency

△ Elderly patients:
- affective disorders
- decreased interest in food
- unusual safety risks
- early stages of dementia
  * very high risk because they are aware of their growing deficits
- substance abuse
- misuse of prescribed medications
- refusal of medical interventions

4. High-risk factors for suicidal behavior:
△ adolescent
△ male
△ Caucasian
△ socially isolated
△ depression
△ hallucinations or delusions
△ intoxication
△ inadequate support system
△ chronically or terminally ill
△ has an established suicide plan
△ prior suicide attempt
△ high-risk professions:
- physicians
- police officers
- attorneys
- dentists
- air-traffic controllers
- military personnel

△ older than 45 years
△ separated, divorced, or widowed
△ chemically dependent
△ student
△ coming out of a depressive state

Δ unemployed

Δ schizophrenic

Δ major life changes (job, family, etc.)

Δ major loss (health, spouse, etc.)

Δ intends shooting, hanging, jumping

Δ family history of suicide attempt

Interventions

1. Complete primary and secondary survey with interventions as indicated.
2. Assess for patient safety and assign patient to treatment area as necessary.
3. Perform specific interventions based on injury inflicted.
   Δ gun shot wound, ingestion, and so on.
4. Arrange for 1:1 observation.
5. Initiate crisis intervention.
6. Obtain lab work as ordered, including appropriate toxicology screens.
7. If you suspect that a depressed patient may be suicidal, ask:
   Δ "Sometimes when people feel this depressed/hopeless/sad, they have thoughts of hurting or killing themselves. Have you ever had thoughts like this?"
   Δ If the patients answers "yes," then assess the following:
   - Does the person have a plan?
   - Assess lethality of plan (handful of aspirin versus a gun).
   - Does person have the means to carry out the plan?
   - Does the person have access to a gun, poison, car, and so on?
   - Has person ever attempted suicide before?

> **ALERT** *Remember:* You **must** take every suicidal gesture *seriously!*

■ DON'T LET THIS BE YOU

She put on her new blue nightgown and combed her hair.
Painted her eyes and her mouth.
Used some Christmas cologne and then she swallowed the pills.

When they brought her to us,
Her gown was soiled and twisted around her body.
Her hair was damp and knotted.
The cosmetics grotesquely smeared on her tear-wet face.
She could still talk.
She took few enough pills for that:
"Let me alone, let me sleep."

We didn't have time to sympathize,
There was a man on the pacemaker in the next room.
A child had died an hour ago.
It was Sunday, too, and naturally we were short of help.
She was, frankly, a nuisance.

The resident passed the slender plastic tube
While she wept and fought, and we held her down.
The new nurse said, "Poor thing . . ."
I said, "Poor thing, nothing. If they're going to do it,
I wish they'd do it right and save us all this bother."
I didn't know she heard me. Maybe I didn't care.

That must have been a month ago.
Tonight she came in again,
D.O.A.
This time she'd hanged herself.
The way I knew her was the same blue nightgown—her face had changed.
The police found a note.
All it said was, "This time I'll do it right."

Only a couple of hours till midnight.
I'll be glad to finish up and go home.
I'm tired as usual and though it's warm in here,
I'm cold and not as unshaken as they think.
I know why I'm cold.
Death touched me again tonight.

Don't worry, I'm not going to brood about it.
It couldn't help her and I know it wouldn't me.
You can't go back.
You can't take back the words,
But I would if I could,
If only I could . . .
This once.

Author unknown.
(Shives, 1990)

OBSTETRICAL ISSUES

General Issues

Common terms:
- Δ Gravidity: Number of times a woman has been pregnant
- Δ Parity: Number of pregnancies resulting in the birth of a viable fetus
- Δ First trimester: First 12 weeks of pregnancy
- Δ Second trimester: 13–26 weeks of pregnancy
- Δ Third trimester: 26 weeks until delivery

Assessment

A. Obtain basic triage assessment per protocol.
B. Perform nursing assessment of the pregnant patient.
   1. Common signs and symptoms:
      - Δ nausea
      - Δ vomiting
      - Δ edema
      - Δ rectal pain
      - Δ fatigue
      - Δ fever
      - Δ syncope
      - Δ headache
      - Δ blurred vision
      - Δ sudden weight gain
      - Δ abdominal cramping
      - Δ hypertension
   2. Past medical history:
      - Δ cardiac disease
      - Δ pulmonary disease
      - Δ renal disease
      - Δ hypertension
      - Δ diabetes
      - Δ thyroid disorders
      - Δ seizure disorder
      - Δ previous obstetrical history
      - Δ date of last normal menstrual cycle
      - Δ estimated date of confinement
      - Δ vaginal bleeding (color, amount, tissue)
      - Δ chemical dependency
      - Δ prenatal care

C. Auscultate for fetal heart tones (FHT):

Using a fetal doppler, fetal heart rate can be assessed as early as 9–12 weeks gestation. FHT can be detected by ultrasound at 6–8 weeks gestation.

1. Technique:

Δ Using the doppler, locate and count the fetal heart rate.

Δ Verify what the mother's heart rate is at that same time.

Δ If the mother is having contractions:

- listen before the contraction, to obtain a baseline FHT
- listen during the contraction
- listen 1 minute after the contraction finishes

2. Interpretations of FHT:

Δ Baseline rate is the average rate occurring between contractions. Normal is 120–160 beats per minute (bpm).

Δ Mild bradycardia is when the baseline rate 100–119 bpm.

Δ Marked bradycardia is a baseline rate <99 bpm.

- **This is cause for serious concern and immediate attention.**

Δ Tachycardia is a persistent baseline rate >180 bpm.

- may occur with maternal fever, drug ingestion, thyrotoxicosis
- may occur with fetal infection or anemia

D. Time uterine contractions:

1. Count from the beginning of one contraction to the beginning of the next contraction (as perceived by the mother or palpated by the nurse).

2. Note how long each contraction lasts, and the interval of the contractions.

3. Count a series of contractions, as they may be irregularly spaced.

Spontaneous Abortion

Δ The termination of pregnancy prior to fetal viability.

Δ Delivery of the fetus before 20 weeks gestation.

Δ Lay public freely uses the term *abortion* to indicate one that is an induced abortion.

Δ *Miscarriage* is the term used by the general population to indicate a spontaneous abortion.

- Health care personnel should be sensitive to the lay person's use of terms.

Δ Parents should be counseled regarding their loss and the grieving that will take place.

Δ Six classifications as listed in the following:

Assessment

	Spontaneous Abortion					
Type	*Signs and Symptoms*	*Uterine Cramping*	*Bleeding*	*Passage of Tissue*	*Internal Cervical Os*	*Possible Management*
Threatened	Low back pain Uterine tenderness	Menstrual-like cramps	Slight	No	Closed	Bedrest
Inevitable	Uterus enlarged and boggy	Moderate	Moderate	No	Open	D&C
Incomplete	Possible hypovol-emic shock Uterus enlarged and boggy Uterus smaller than expected for dates	Severe	Heavy	Yes	Open with tissue in the os	D&C
Complete	Uterus small and nontender	Mild	Scant	Yes	Closed	Variable
Septic	Fever Malodorous vagi-nal bleeding Uterus extremely tender on palpa-tion	Variable	Variable	Variable	Open	D&C Antibiotics Maintain ABCs
Missed	History of missed menses Uterus smaller than expected for dates Ultrasound shows intrauterine pro-ducts of concep-tion without heart beat	No	Slight	No	Closed	Fetal delivery

(Reminton-Klein, 1994; Kitt, 1995; Sinclair, 1996)

Interventions

1. Dependent on type of loss
2. May need IV access for administration of fluids and/or medications
3. Rh coagulation profile (administration of RhoGAM if woman is Rh negative)
4. Provide emotional care for grieving woman and family

Ectopic Pregnancy

Δ The implantation of the fertilized ovum outside the uterine cavity.
Δ 96% of ectopic implantations occur in the fallopian tubes.

ALERT   Vaginal bleeding and abdominal pain in a reproductive-age female signify an ectopic pregnancy **until proven otherwise.**

Assessment

1. History:
   Δ pelvic inflammatory disease
   Δ congenital or developmental anomalies of the fallopian tube(s)
   Δ previous ectopic pregnancy
   Δ tubal ligation
   Δ use of an intrauterine device
   Δ infertility
   Δ multiple induced abortions
   Δ pelvic inflammatory disease (PID)
   Δ endometriosis
2. Common signs and symptoms:
   Δ sudden, severe pelvic pain
   Δ nausea and vomiting
   Δ syncope
   Δ cervical motion tenderness
   Δ enlarged uterus
   Δ amenorrhea (average, 5.5 weeks)
   Δ 1–2 days of vaginal spotting
   Δ positive orthostatic vital signs
   Δ abdominal pain on palpation
   Δ tachycardia and hypotension
3. Abnormal lab values:
   Δ WBC elevated
   Δ scrum qualitative hCG positive
   Δ decreased hemoglobin and hematocrit

Interventions

1. Maintain ABCs.
2. Monitor vital signs closely.
3. Place one or two large-bore intravenous lines; rate depends on hemodynamic status.

4. Type and cross as indicated for transfusion.
5. Provide patient support and education for loss of pregnancy, and preoperative preparation.
6. Administer Rh immunoglobulin to all Rh negative patients.

Placenta Previa

Δ Placenta is abnormally implanted in the lower uterine segment, to some degree occluding the cervical os.

Assessment

1. Common signs and symptoms:
   Δ **painless** vaginal bleeding occurring 28–32 weeks gestation
   Δ bright red vaginal bleeding
   Δ FHTs may show ominous patterns
   Δ ultrasound shows placenta over cervical os

Interventions

1. *Do not perform a vaginal examination* (can cause fatal hemorrhage).
2. Maintain ABCs.
3. Position mother on her left side (displaces the uterus off the inferior vena cava).
4. Type and cross as indicated for transfusion.
5. Establish and maintain large bore intravenous line(s).
6. Monitor vital signs of mother and fetal heart tones closely.
7. Assess CBC, coagulation studies, and Rh antibody status.

Abruptio Placentae

Δ Accidental hemorrhage caused by the separation of the normally located placenta before delivery of the fetus.

Assessment

1. History:
   Δ essential hypertension
   Δ multiple gestation
   Δ external trauma
   Δ smoking
   Δ uterine fibroids
   Δ pregnancy-induced hypertension

Δ previous abruptio placentae or placenta previa
Δ substance abuse (especially cocaine)
Δ preterm premature rupture of membranes
Δ advanced maternal age

2. Common signs and symptoms:
   Δ tender, rigid uterus
   Δ fetal distress
   Δ **painful** vaginal bleeding
   Δ vaginal bleeding may be absent
   • if encapsulated by placenta or membranes

3. Complications:
   Δ fetal death
   Δ renal failure
   Δ hypovolemic shock
   Δ disseminated intravascular coagulation (DIC)

 Interventions

1. Maintain ABCs.
2. Do not perform a vaginal examination until placenta previa is ruled out.
3. Monitor maternal vital signs and fetal heart rate closely.
4. Place large bore intravenous line(s).
5. Position mother on her left side (displaces uterus off the inferior vena cava).
6. Type and cross as indicated for transfusion.
7. Assess CBC, Rh status, coagulation studies, toxicology screen.
8. Prepare for possibility of emergency delivery.

Pre-eclampsia and Eclampsia

Δ These complications of pregnancy-induced hypertension are the leading cause of maternal death in the United States.

 Assessment

1. Characteristic symptoms:
   Δ onset of symptoms from the 20th week of gestation to 1–10 days postpartum
   Δ hypertension
   • positive pregestational history of hypertension, compare current BP with patient's normal BP
   • negative history of pregestional hypertension, then hypertension is considered anything above a systolic BP >120 or diastolic BP >80–90 mmHg

Δ proteinuria (300 mg or more of protein excreted in a 24-hour period)

Δ nondependent edema, present after 8–12 hours of bedrest (face, fingers, body)

Δ weight gain >2 lb in 1 week, or 6 lb in 1 month

2. Severe pre-eclampsia will have additional symptoms:

Δ systolic BP >160 mmHg

Δ oliguria

Δ severe headache

Δ pulmonary edema

Δ hyperreflexia

Δ serum creatinine >1.2 mg/dL

Δ retinal hemorrhages

Δ decreased fribinogen level

Δ diastolic BP >110 mmHg

Δ proteinuria (>5 g/24 hr sample)

Δ visual changes (blurring, double vision)

Δ thrombocytopenia (platelet count <100,000)

Δ intrauterine growth retardation

Δ increased liver enzymes

Δ papilledema

Δ epigastric pain (indicative of hepatic hemorrhage)

3. Eclampsia occurs when the central nervous system is so influenced by vasospasm that seizures develop.

Interventions (depend on the severity of the disease and symptoms)

1. Maintain ABCs.
2. Monitor maternal vital signs and FHT closely.
3. Establish intravenous access site(s) for medication administration.
4. Initiate a conservative rate with crystalloid fluid rate *no greater than* 100 mL/hr.
5. Strictly record intake and output.
6. Place foley catheter.
7. Administer magnesium sulfate ($MgSO_4$) to prevent and treat convulsions

Δ loading dose of 3–4 g

Δ continual $MgSO_4$ IV drip dose of 1–4 g/hr

Δ may be given IM if IV access not immediately available

8. Prepare for immediate delivery if patient's condition worsens.

Gestational Diabetes Mellitus

Δ May occur in previously nondiabetic women as a result of metabolic changes.

Assessment

1. History:
   - Δ stillbirth
   - Δ hydramnios
   - Δ maternal obesity
   - Δ hypertension
   - Δ infant with congenital anomalies
   - Δ infant weight >9 lbs
   - Δ family history of diabetes
   - Δ maternal age >35
2. Effects of diabetes on:
   - Δ mother
     - increased risk of pregnancy-induced hypertension
     - infections that may be more severe
     - birth trauma owing to increased fetal size
     - postpartum hemorrhage
   - Δ fetus
     - faulty DNA and RNA synthesis, resulting in congenital anomalies
     - delayed lung maturity
     - increased fetal growth rate
     - after birth, neonatal hypoglycemia
3. Common symptoms:
   - Δ polyuria
   - Δ polydipsia
   - Δ glucosuria
   - Δ chronic monilial infection
   - Δ polyphagia
   - Δ weight loss
   - Δ urine positive for ketones
4. Laboratory values:
   - Δ elevated serum glucose levels at 24–28 weeks (>125 mg/dL)
   - Δ elevated serum glucose challenge test

 Interventions

1. Stabilize serum glucose level.
2. Provide patient education, including:
   - Δ facts about gestational diabetes
   - Δ nutritional counseling
   - Δ exercise
3. Close follow-up with primary care provider if patient discharged.

Premature Rupture of Membranes

Δ The spontaneous rupture of amniotic membranes prior to the onset of labor regardless of gestational age.

Assessment

1. History:
   Δ multiple gestations
   Δ breech presentations
   Δ chorioamnionitis
   Δ fetal distress
2. Common signs and symptoms:
   Δ fluid from vagina, in varying amounts
3. Complications:
   Δ amnionitis
   Δ endometritis
   Δ asphyxia
   Δ prematurity
   Δ cord prolapse
   Δ fetal injuries secondary to low amniotic fluid volume
   Δ malpresentation
   Δ respiratory distress
   Δ cord compression

Interventions (dependent on gestational age and if labor has begun)

1. Monitor vitals signs and FHR.
2. Perform sterile speculum exam.
   Δ assess for cervical effacement and dilation
   Δ evaluate fluid from the posterior vaginal vault using litmus or nitrazine paper
   • amniotic fluid is alkaline, and will turn litmus or nitrazine paper blue
   • blood can give a false-positive nitrazine test
   • microscopic evaluation of dried fluid for a ferning pattern
   • blood or other secretions can produce a false-negative ferning test
   Δ if fluid leakage is intermittent, nitrazine, litmus, and ferning exams may be inconclusive for intact membranes
   Δ evaluate for a prolapsed umbilical cord
3. Defer bimanual examination until labor is active.
4. Establish and maintain large-bore intravenous line(s).

Preterm Labor

Δ Occurs 20–37 weeks of gestation and produces cervical changes.

 Assessment

1. History
   Δ infection
   Δ fetal abnormalities
   Δ multiple gestation
   Δ cerclage
   Δ cocaine use
   Δ abortion
   Δ trauma
   Δ poor nutritional status
   Δ emotional stress
   Δ maternal fever or sepsis
   Δ maternal diabetes
   Δ diethylstilbestrol (DES) exposure in utero
     • DES caused cervical anomalies and incompetence
   Δ uterine anomalies
   Δ previous cervical conization
   Δ previous preterm birth
   Δ abdominal surgery during this pregnancy
   Δ maternal age <18 or >35 years
   Δ absent or inadequate prenatal care
   Δ more than 10 cigarettes smoked in a day
   Δ second or third trimester bleeding
2. Common signs and symptoms:
   Δ menstrual cramps
   Δ back discomfort
   Δ vaginal pain
   Δ abdominal pain or discomfort
   Δ change in vaginal discharge
   Δ pelvic, rectal, or bladder pressure

 Interventions

1. Monitor maternal vital signs and FHR.
2. Time several contractions when possible.
3. Perform sterile speculum exam, as stated for PROM.
4. Perform gentle bimanual exam if membranes *are not* ruptured.

5. Establish large-bore intravenous line(s).
6. Arrange for transfer to labor and delivery unit and for fetal monitoring.

Trauma in Pregnancy

Δ Fetal survival depends on the integrity of the woman's condition and stability.
Δ Initially, all efforts should be centered on stabilization and treatment of the woman, with subsequent evaluation and treatment of the unborn child.

Assessment

1. History:
   Δ fall
   Δ physical assault
   Δ motor vehicle crash
2. Primary and secondary assessments as indicated for *all* trauma victims.
3. Uterine activity, including:
   Δ tenderness or contractions
   Δ cervical dilation
   Δ vaginal bleeding
   Δ umbilical cord prolapse
   Δ ruptured membranes
4. Fetal distress:
   Δ fetal heart tones
   Δ fetal movement
   Δ fetal monitoring

Interventions

1. Maintain ABCs.
2. Immobilize the c-spine.
3. Refer to Multiple Trauma Guideline.
4. If no c-spine injury, place woman on her left side to prevent inferior vena cava compression and hypotension. If woman has a spinal injury, log roll patient on the spinal board and support board with rolled towels under it, to maintain patient on her left side.
5. Anticipate hypovolemia and treat blood loss aggressively.
6. CT scans are often suggested, as plain films of the abdomen may be distorted.
7. A pediatrician and an obstetrician should be mobilized to the ED for evaluation and preparation for possible emergency delivery.
8. Administer tetanus prophylaxis per protocol.
9. Transfer to obstetrical unit on stabilization.

Emergency Delivery

Δ Optimally, childbirth should occur in the labor and delivery department of a hospital. On rare occasions, however, a woman will deliver prior to arriving in the obstetrical department.

Δ The ED staff must be prepared to care for the mother and baby in this situation.

 Assessment

1. Signs of Imminent Delivery:
   Δ increased bloody show
   Δ contractions every 2–3 minutes
   Δ involuntary pushing
   Δ perineal and rectal flattening
   Δ crowning of the fetal scalp at the introitus
   Δ rectal pressure or passage of feces
   Δ mother states "the baby is coming"
   Δ spontaneous rupture of membranes
   Δ bulging of the perineum

ALERT If delivery is imminent, do *not* attempt to transport patient. Prepare for a controlled delivery in the ED.

 Interventions

1. Obtain necessary equipment:
   Δ two cord clamps
   Δ sterile scissors
   Δ protective gloves, masks, gowns
   Δ neonatal resuscitative equipment
   Δ hemostats
   Δ ample linen
   Δ suction
2. Obtain isolette or warmed blankets for newborn.
3. Continually care for the mother until delivery of the placenta; observe for hemorrhage.
4. Assess Apgar score for infant at 1 and 5 minutes.
5. Document important information:
   Δ time of birth
   Δ type of presentation
   Δ cord around neck?
   Δ time of membrane rupture
   Δ time of placenta delivery
   Δ Apgar scores at 1 and 5 minutes

APGAR Scoring Chart

	Sign	0	1	2	1 Minute Score	5 Minute Score
A	Appearance (color)	Blue or pale	Pink body with blue extremities	Completely pink		
P	Pulse (heart rate)	Absent	Slow (<100)	>100		
G	Grimace (reflexes)	No response	Facial grimace	Cough, sneeze, crying		
A	Activity (muscle tone)	Limp	Some flexion	Active motion		
R	Respirations	Absent	Slow, irregular (weak cry)	Good (vigorous crying)		

ORTHOPAEDIC INJURIES (GENERAL)

 Assessment

A. Obtain and record triage assessment:
   - Δ mechanism of injury
   - Δ time of injury
   - Δ immediate care of injured extremity (splinted, walked on it, etc.)
   - Δ possibility of other injuries.
B. Assess injured area for:
   - Δ obvious deformity (angulation, rotation, shortening, etc.)
   - Δ swelling
   - Δ pain (at rest, with movement, on palpation, etc.)
   - Δ decreased sensation
   - Δ partial or complete loss of motor function
   - Δ skin coolness or blanching
   - Δ quality of pulses distal to the injury
C. Complete remainder of basic triage assessment, and *document* accurately.

 Immediate Care If:

Δ Open fracture:
   - notify ED physician immediately
   - aseptically control bleeding
   - cover open wound with sterile gauze
   - arrange for stabilization of the injury
Δ Closed fracture that is:
   - unstable
   - alteration in circulation distal to injury
   - advise ED physician of patient status

 Interventions

1. Remove *all* rings from *all* fingers with hand, wrist, or forearm injuries.
2. If closed injury with possibility of a fracture:
   - Δ reassure patient
   - Δ apply splint to increase patient comfort and decrease risk of further injury
   - Δ apply ice and elevate extremity
3. If triage nurse anticipates the need for an x-ray:
   - Δ follow departmental policy with regard to ordering x-ray study from triage

COMMON FRACTURES

The triage nurse should possess a basic understanding of the most common fractures. Doing so enhances the nurse's ability to prioritize the patient's acuity and provide initial nursing care of the patient.

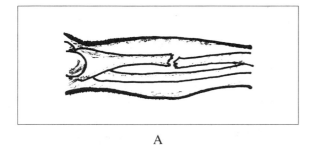

A

Simple Fracture

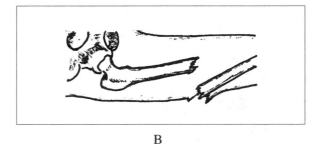

B

Compound Fracture (open)

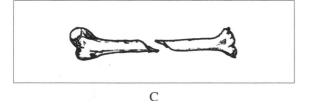

C

Spiral Fracture

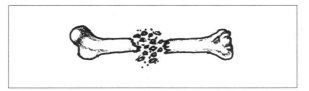

D

Comminuted Fracture

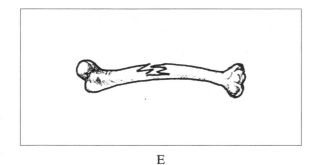

E

Greenstick Fracture

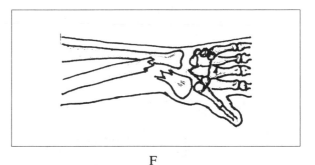

F

Colles' Fracture

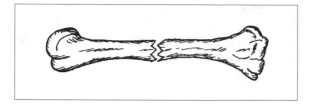

G

Transverse Fracture

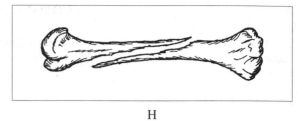

H

Longitudinal Fracture

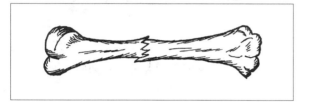

I

Impacted Fracture

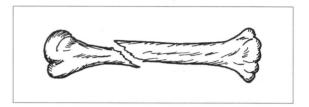

J

Oblique Fracture

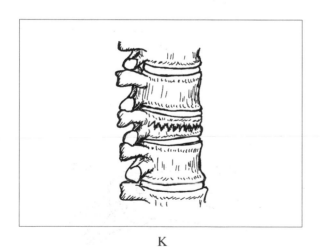

K

Spinal Compression Fracture

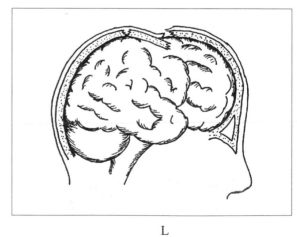

L

Depressed Skull Fracture

RASH

Δ A broad term used to describe a dermatologic manifestation that may include hives, infections (fungal, viral, bacterial), insect bites, or contact dermatitis.

Δ Rashes may be primary, secondary, vascular, or contagious in nature.

Δ It is *vital* for the nurse to be able to properly document the lesions and to identify those that may be contagious.

Δ When inspecting the skin, be sure to have:
- adequate lighting
- tape measure to assist in assessing the size of the lesions.

Δ Patient privacy should be maintained during this evaluation.

Δ Always wear gloves when assessing a rash or skin lesion.

General Issues

Assessment

A. Obtain and record telephone triage assessment:
  1. History of allergies:
     Δ prior exposures, reactions, or anaphylaxis
     Δ new products or medications
  2. Characteristics of rash:
     Δ location
       - localized
       - widespread
       - area of the body
     Δ size
       - approximate size of lesions
     Δ shape
       - linear
       - circular
       - grouped
       - scattered
       - generalized
       - diffuse
     Δ color
       - pink
       - red
       - purple
       - yellow
       - brown
       - green
     Δ consistency
       - flat or smooth
       - raised or bumpy

- hard or soft
- firm
Δ temperature
- cool
- warm
- hot to touch
Δ mobility
- fixed
- movable masses
- fluid filled
- open
- draining
Δ signs of infection
- redness
- swelling
- red streaks
- warm to touch

3. Associated symptoms and behavior:
Δ fever
Δ headache
Δ drowsiness
Δ facial or eye swelling
Δ "cold" symptoms
Δ itching
Δ sore throat
Δ joint pain
Δ vision changes
Δ refusal or inability to swallow
Δ nausea, vomiting, or diarrhea
Δ swollen glands

B. Assess for risk factors that may increase the acuity of a rash:
Δ Prior allergic reaction
Δ Chronic illness
Δ Immunosuppressed (congenital, acquired, or chemically induced)

Immediate Care If

Δ difficulty breathing, wheezing, and/or chest tightness
Δ recent exposure to possible or known toxin with development of:
- cough
- slurred speech or hoarseness
- swollen tongue or difficulty swallowing

Δ wheezing after ingestion of medication, allergic food, or bee sting
  • use prescribed anaphylactic kit as directed for known allergies
Δ purple or blood-colored spots with or without a fever
Δ fever greater than 105°F
Δ bright red skin that peels off in sheets
Δ severe headache with a fever >100°F
Δ hives began <2 hours ago and has had severe allergic reaction in the past

Primary Lesions

Assessment

Δ Primary lesions arise from previously normal skin and are described as:

Macule = Flat, nonpalpable, discolored, <1 cm (e.g., freckle, drug rash, measles, scarlet fever)
Papule = Elevated, solid lesion <1 cm (e.g., wart, raised scaly area of psoriasis, small bug bite, pityriasis rosea)
Plaque = Like a macule or papule, but >1 cm in diameter (e.g., birthmark, mongolian spot, plantar wart, psoriasis, pityriasis rosea)
Nodule = Elevated, solid lesion 1–2 cm in diameter, moves with skin when palpated (e.g., ganglion, area of poorly absorbed injection)

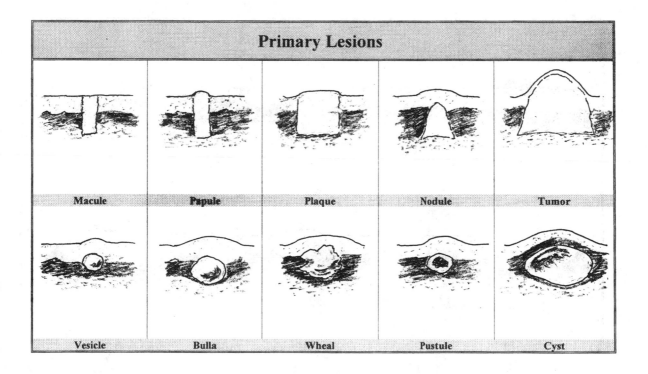

Primary Lesions

| Macule | Papule | Plaque | Nodule | Tumor |
| Vesicle | Bulla | Wheal | Pustule | Cyst |

Tumor = Elevated, solid lesion >2 cm, may be soft or firm (e.g., tumor of any type)

Vesicle = Elevated lesion <1 cm filled with clear fluid (e.g., blister, chickenpox, poison ivy, herpes simplex, herpes zoster)

Bulla = Elevated lesion >1 cm filled with clear fluid (e.g., bullous impetigo, on hands or feet with syphilis, poison ivy, burns)

Pustule = Elevated, pus-filled lesion (e.g., acne, impetigo, boil)

Wheal = Elevated lesion with circumscribed pink borders and light center (e.g., hives, urticaria, insect bite, poison sumac, poison ivy)

Cyst = Encapsulated, fluid-filled area in the dermis or subcutaneous tissue (e.g., sebaceous cyst, epidermoid cyst)

Secondary Lesions

 Assessment

Δ Secondary lesions usually begin as a primary change or lesion in the skin.

Crust = Dried serum or blood exudate (e.g., abrasion, ruptured blisters)

Scar = Connective tissue formed during the healing process that replaces skin damaged to the depth of the dermis (e.g., hypertrophied, atrophied, keloid)

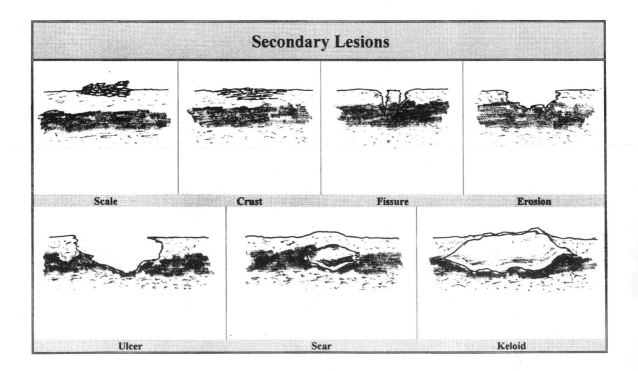

Secondary Lesions

Scale · Crust · Fissure · Erosion

Ulcer · Scar · Keloid

Fissure = Linear crack in epidermis (e.g., chapping, cracked lips as seen with dehydration, exposure, fever)

Erosion = Depressed, moist surface change affecting the epidermis (e.g., superficial scratch, syphilitic chancre, broken chickenpox vesicle)

Ulcer = Necrotic hollowing of epidermis and dermis (e.g., decubiti)

Scale = A flake of dead epithelium (e.g., psoriasis, seborrheic dermatitis, exfoliative dermatitis)

Keloid = Overproduction of scar tissue that appears raised, red, and smooth (e.g., high incidence of occurrence in African Americans)

Vascular Lesions

Assessment

Δ Indicate trauma or systemic problems such as:
- clotting disorders
- leukemia
- infectious processes

Ecchymoses = Discoloration; various shades of red; yellow as time since onset increases; variable size (e.g., trauma, septicemia, hepatic dysfunction, bleeding disorders)

Hematoma = Reddish purple or skin-toned, elevated, variable in size. Results from the collection of extravasated blood contained in the tissues of the skin (e.g., trauma, incomplete hemostasis after invasive procedure/surgery)

Petechiae = Reddish-purple spots <0.5 cm, result from capillary bleeding, do not blanch (e.g., leukemia, inadequate or defective platelets, bacterial endocarditis)

Purpura = Reddish-purple spots >0.5 cm, do not blanch (e.g., thrombocytopenic purpura, intravascular defects, infection)

Spider angioma = Bright-red center with radiating lines, blanches, usually found on face, neck, shoulders, upper chest (e.g., liver dysfunction, vitamin B deficiency, pregnancy)

Cherry angioma = Bright-red, round lesions that may brown with age (e.g., nonpathologic and occur with normal aging process)

Telangiectasia = Dilation of capillaries and thinning of vascular walls that appear as bluish lines on the face and/or thighs (e.g., alcoholism, polycythemia, disorders with bleeding tendency)

Venous star = Bluish areas that will not blanch and usually occur on legs or chest (e.g., increased pressure on superficial veins, distention, activity)

Contagious Rashes

△ Pose the risk of spreading infection to other individuals in the Emergency Department.

△ It is important for the triage nurse to be able to identify these rashes, and *appropriately isolate the patient directly from triage.*

 Assessment

The following are potentially contagious rashes:

Potentially Contagious Rashes		
Problem	*Characteristics*	*Associated Signs and Symptoms*
Measles	Generalized, papular, red red, blotchy rash	Koplik's spots in mouth, runny nose, light sensitivity, fever, pruritus, cough
Chicken pox (varicella)	Vesicular with crusting lesions in various stages; generalized	Runny nose, fever, cough, pruritus
	Rash lesions are maculopapular for a few hours, vesicular for 3–4 days, and then leave a scab	
Impetigo	Vesicular with crusting over erythematous base; localized initially, then spreading	
Scabies	Papules, vesicles, or linear rash often between fingers, on neck, and on forearms, but may be atypical	Severe, persistent pruritus

SYNCOPE

Assessment

A. Obtain triage assessment that includes:
   1. History:
      Δ visual changes
      Δ altered mental status
      Δ recent infections
      Δ chemical dependency
      Δ recent exercise
      Δ diet changes
      Δ known trauma
      Δ facial numbness
      Δ chemical or environmental exposure
      Δ medications (prescription and OTC)
      Δ medical conditions:
         • cardiac
         • neurologic
         • pregnancy
         • endocrine
   2. Associated signs and symptoms:
      Δ dizziness
      Δ pallor
      Δ palpitations
      Δ malaise
      Δ weakness
      Δ ataxia
      Δ unsteady gait
      Δ speech irregularities
      Δ visual changes
      Δ vomiting
      Δ sudden, severe headache
      Δ irregular heart beat
      Δ positive orthostatic vital signs
      Δ pupillary response abnormality
      Δ unequal hand grasps
      Δ altered mentation
      Δ numbness of face, arm, leg

Immediate Care If

Δ unstable vital signs
Δ positive orthostatic vital signs
Δ cardiac arrhythmias
Δ blood loss
Δ warning signs of stroke
  • weakness or numbness
    * face
    * arm
    * leg
    * one side of body
  • visual changes (especially unilateral)
    * sudden dimness
    * blurring
    * decreased sight
  • speech disturbances
    * loss of language
    * difficulty talking
    * difficulty understanding conversation
  • unexplained dizziness, vertigo, or decreased coordination
  • sudden severe headache

 Interventions

1. Provide for patient safety.
2. Maintain ABCs.

TRAUMA, MULTIPLE (ADULT)

Any victim of trauma will be evaluated and treated according to your hospital's ED Trauma Protocol. The following is a brief outline of the sequenced events that will occur. The ED team will *need to adjust* the protocol to meet the *individual needs* of each trauma victim.

A When notification of an incoming trauma victim is received, the ED charge/triage nurse must immediately:

1. Communicate to appropriate personnel
   - Δ MD
   - Δ supervisor
   - Δ ED staff
   - Δ ancillary services
     - operating room
     - registration
     - laboratory
     - trauma or code team as needed
     - respiratory therapy
     - radiology
     - EKG

2. Assign staff who will care for other ED patients.

3. Prepare trauma room, verify available setup of:
   - Δ oxygen (nonrebreather mask and ambu-bag ready)
   - Δ suction (consider two setups)
   - Δ cardiac monitor in "on" position
   - Δ position BP machine, oximeter, and thermometer at bedside
   - Δ IV solutions, tubing, supplies
   - Δ open appropriate cart if need indicates
   - Δ critical care flow sheet for documentation
   - Δ universal precaution protection equipment
   - Δ assign staff roles in trauma care (documentation, IV, meds, etc.)

B. When patient arrives, the ED team will:

1. Obtain brief report from Emergency Medical Service (EMS) crew.

2. Assist with patient transfer from EMS stretcher onto trauma stretcher *while maintaining c-spine and airway precautions.*

C. Perform primary survey and intervene immediately as necessary:

1. Airway with c-spine control
   - Δ clear and open airway
     - administer oxygen by mask
   - Δ partially or potentially obstructed airway:
     - clear obstruction if possible, carefully observe, administer oxygen
   - Δ obstructed airway:
     - prepare for intubation or crichothyrotomy

2. Breathing:
   - Δ assess rate, depth, regularity, and ease of respiratory effort
   - Δ assess for use of accessory and abdominal muscles

Δ assess for chest wall integrity and symmetry of expansion
Δ assess for decreased level of consciousness
Δ assess for cyanosis

3. Circulation:
Δ assess pulse quality, location and rate
- if *radial* pulse is present, systolic BP is at least 80 mmHg
- if *femoral* pulse is present, systolic BP is at least 70 mmHg
- if *carotid* pulse is present, systolic BP is at least 60 mmHg

Δ place patient on cardiac monitor, run a strip
Δ assess capillary refill (normal is 1–2 sec)
Δ assess skin color
Δ note obvious sources of bleeding
Δ assess level of consciousness
Δ apply BP cuff (manual or machine)
Δ apply oximetry probe, correlate pulse to verify O_2% reading
Δ insert IVs as indicated, usually two large-bore catheters (14–18 gauge)
Δ obtain blood samples

4. Disability:
Δ assess level of consciousness
Δ obtain subjective data including:
- mechanism of injury
- patient complaints
- areas of pain, numbness, tingling, and ability to move
- treatment at accident scene and prior to arrival
- allergies
- current medications, including anticoagulants, ETOH, or use of illegal drugs
- last tetanus immunization
- past medical and surgical history
- any family, friends, or clergy the patient wants called

5. Expose and examine:
Δ undress the patient completely
Δ provide for warmth and privacy of patient
Δ assess neurological status completely

D. Perform secondary survey and intervene as necessary.
Once the quick primary survey is completed and life-threatening problems have been attended to, the ED team progresses to systematically performing a thorough assessment of the patient. Careful documentation is essential.

1. Obtain complete set of vital signs.
2. Assess general appearance.
Δ body positioning
Δ guarding
Δ body posture
Δ self-protection movements
3. Note any odors
Δ gasoline

Δ urine

Δ feces

Δ alcohol

Δ chemical odors

Δ anything unusual

4. Perform head-to-toe assessment, checking for symmetry, deformity, discomfort, swelling, bleeding, and depression.

Δ head and face
- bone deformities
- soft tissue injuries

Δ neck
- inspect
- palpate

Δ clavicles and chest
- bony deformities
- soft tissue injury
- expansion during ventilation
- observe and auscaltate breathing

Δ abdomen
- distention
- bruising
- soft tissue injury
- auscaltate bowel sounds
- palpate all four quadrants

Δ pelvis and genitalia
- soft tissue injury
- place hands on each side of the pelvis, and gently squeeze inward to assess for tenderness, crepitus, instability
- bleeding from the urethral meatus
- rectal exam by the physician should always be performed *prior* to the placement of the foley catheter

Δ extremities
- soft tissue injury
- sensory function
- bony deformity
- motor function
- circulatory status
- crepitus

Δ posterior assessment
- maintain c-spine precautions
- assist MD in log rolling patient, utilizing ED team

Glasgow Coma Scale

The Glasgow Coma Scale (GCS) is a method of quantifying a patient's state of consciousness. It is an assessment tool used for patients with trauma, head injuries, headaches, etc. The accuracy of the GCS may be affected if the patient is hypoxic or hypotensive. It is important to use the GCS as a *part* of the patient's total assessment.

Glasgow Coma Scale				
	Infant (Preverbal)		*Child/Adult*	
Eye opening	4	Spontaneously	4	Spontaneously
	3	To speech	3	To voice command or speech
	2	To pain	2	To pain
	1	No response	1	No response
Best verbal response	5	Coos/babbles/cries appropriately	5	Oriented
	4	Irritable cry	4	Confused
	3	Cries only to pain	3	Inappropriate words
	2	Moans or grunts to pain	2	Incomprehensible words or vocal sounds
	1	No response	1	No response
Best motor response	6	Spontaneous	6	Obeys commands
	5	Localizes pain or withdraws to touch	5	Localizes pain, purposeful movements
	4	Withdraws from pain	4	Withdraws from pain
	3	Abnormal flexion to pain (decorticate)	3	Abnormal flexion to pain (decorticate)
	2	Abnormal extension to pain (decerebrate)	2	Abnormal extension to pain (decerebrate)
	1	No response	1	No response
Total Score =				

Trauma Score

△ This is an important field index that assists health care professionals in assessing the severity of the patient's injury.

△ The trauma score should be used on patients who do *not* have an obvious head injury.

△ This tool assesses respiratory rate, respiratory effort, systolic blood pressure, capillary refill, and the GCS.

△ A number is assigned to each finding and the total score is between 1 and 16.

△ A trauma score of 16 predicts a 99% survival rate, whereas a trauma score of 1 predicts a 0% survival rate (Miller, 1996).

△ A score of less than 12 should be considered for immediate transfer to a level I trauma center.

Trauma Score

Physical Sign	Value	Points
Respiratory rate	10–24	4
	25–35	3
	>35	2
	<10	1
	0	0
Respiratory effort	Normal	1
	Shallow or retractive	0
Systolic blood pressure	>90	4
	70–89	3
	50–69	2
	<50	1
	0	0
Capillary refill	1–2 sec (normal)	2
	>3 sec (delayed)	1
	None	0
Glasgow coma scale	14–15	5
	11–13	4
	8–10	3
	5–7	2
	4	1
	3	0

Estimated Survival Rate Based on Trauma Score

Trauma Score	Survival (%)
16	99
14	96
12	87
10	60
8	26
6	8
4	2
2	0

Revised Trauma Score

Δ The *revised trauma score* (RTS) is similar to the trauma score. It allows more weight to be given to the GCS and a more accurate assessment of the patient with an isolated head injury.

Δ A number is assigned to each finding as follows:

Revised Trauma Score		
Variable	*Value*	*Points*
Glasgow Coma Scale	13–15	4
	9–12	3
	6–8	2
	4–5	1
	3	0
Systolic blood pressure	>89	4
	70–89	3
	50–69	2
	1–49	1
	0	0
Respiratory rate	10–29	4
	>29	3
	6–9	2
	<6	1
	0	0

Estimated Survival Rate Based on Revised Trauma Score	
Revised Trauma Score	*Survival (%)*
12	99
10	88
8	67
6	63
4	33
2	28

The total score will be 1–12, with the estimated survival rate for each above.

Mechanisms of Injury From Trauma: Adult

Trauma	Associated Injuries
Pedestrian struck by car • adult point of impact is usually knee/hip	Fractures of the femur, tibia, and fibula on side of impact Fractured pelvis Contralateral ligament damage to knee
Pedestrian struck by car • short adult/child point of im- pact involves chest and/or head	Contralateral skull fracture Chest injury with rib and/or sternal fracture May be thrown, resulting in head/back injury Shoulder dislocation and/or scapular fracture Patellar and lower femur fracture
Pedestrian dragged under a vehicle	Pelvic fracture
Unrestrained: front seat passenger • front impact	Posterior dislocation of acetabulum Fractures of femurs and/or patellas
Unrestrained: driver • front impact	Head injury, c-spine injury, pelvic fracture Flail chest, fractured sternum Aortic or tracheal tears Pulmonary/cardiac contusion Ruptured or lacerated liver or spleen Femur and/or patellar fracture, hip dislocation
Unrestrained: driver or passenger • side impact	Chest: flail, fractured sternum, pulmonary/cardiac contusion Fractures of clavicle, acetabulum, pelvis Lateral neck strain or injury Driver: ruptured spleen Passenger: ruptured liver
Passenger: without head restraint • rear impact	Hyperextension of neck resulting in high c-spine or vertebral fracture or ruptured disk, causing intradural hemorrhage, edema, cord compression
Rotational force from spinning car	Combination of frontal and side impact–induced injuries
Rollover of vehicle	Multitude of external and internal injuries
Ejection from vehicle	Injuries at point of impact
Restrained: driver or passenger	Compression of soft tissue organs, c-spine injuries, rib and sternal frac- tures, cardiac contusions, ruptured diaphragm Lap belt only: head, neck, facial and chest injuries Shoulder strap only: severe neck injury, decapitation Air bag deployed: facial injuries, abrasions/burns of arms
Fall • landing on feet	Compression fractures of lumbosacral spine Fractures of calcaneus
Fall • landing on buttocks	Compression fracture of lumbar vertebrae Pelvic fracture Coccyx fracture
Diving • head first	Forceful cervical spine compression resulting in fracture, dislocation, and/or vertebral bone fragments displaced into spinal canal

continued

Mechanisms of Injury From Trauma: Adult (Continued)

Blunt head trauma • person's moving head strikes a stationary object	Coup/contracoup injury Depressed skull fracture Cerebral hematoma, contusions, or laceration
Blunt chest trauma • moving object strikes a person's chest	Pulmonary contusion Hemothorax Rib fractures

Crush injury to chest	Traumatic asphyxia
	• crushing trauma to chest forces blood from heart via the superior vena cava to veins of the head, neck, and upper chest, causing:
	  • subconjunctival and retinal hemorrhage
	  • conjunctival edema
	  • characteristic deep violet skin color

(Adapted from Miller, 1997.)

■ TRIAGE QUESTIONS FOR PATIENTS INVOLVED IN A MOTOR VEHICLE ACCIDENT

- When did the accident occur?
  - day
  - time
- Where did it occur?
  - highway
  - country road
  - city street
- Was the patient wearing a seat belt?
  - what type? (lap, shoulder, etc.)
  - effectiveness during the accident?
- What speed was the patient's car traveling?
  - approximate speed of other vehicles involved in accident
- Where was the patient sitting in the car?
  - driver
  - front seat passenger
  - back seat passenger
  - box of the truck
- What kind of vehicle was the patient in?
  - What damage was done to the vehicle?
- Did the airbag deploy?
- Did the patient lose consciousness?
  - for how long?
- What is the last thing the patient remembers *before* the accident?
- What is the first thing the patient remembers *after* the accident?

- How was the patient injured in the car?
  - flying objects within the car?
  - car crushed by other vehicle, tree, pole, etc.?
- Was the patient thrown from the car?
  - Was something in the car thrown against the patient?
- Was the patient ambulatory at the scene?
  - Did the patient need to be extricated from the vehicle?
  - How long did it take?
- Were there any other people in the car?
  - Were they injured?
  - What are their injuries?
- Was the pediatric patient in a car seat?
  - Where was the car seat located within the vehicle?
  - Was it struck by a deployed air bag?
  - Was the car seat strapped tightly with the seatbelt?
- Were there law enforcement personnel at the scene?
  - if so, which agency?
- Does the patient wear:
  - contact lenses?
  - glasses?
  - were they worn at the scene?
  - dentures?
  - female patients: Is a tampon in place?
- Where is the patient experiencing pain?
- Is the patient taking any medication, especially aspirin or other anticoagulants?
- Is there anyone the patient wishes to have notified

(Kitt et al., 1995; Handysides, 1996; Kidd, 1996)

TRAUMA, MULTIPLE (PEDIATRIC)

Δ Pediatric trauma is a life-threatening situation that requires the ED staff to perform quickly and precisely.

Δ The smaller size of pediatric trauma victims predisposes them to a clinical status that can easily deteriorate.

Δ It is therefore essential that
- Quick and accurate injury assessment occurs (consider using the Pediatric Injury Assessment Form).
- Treatment is quickly implemented.
- Transfer to a Pediatric Trauma Center is implemented when appropriate.
- Accurate documentation occurs.

Δ Pediatric patients differ from adult patients in some ways, and it is important for ED nurses to understand those differences and prepare for them accordingly.

ALERT

Δ Children have greater oxygen demands and caloric requirements because of a higher metabolic rate.

Δ Children have highly reactive vascular systems that maintain systolic blood pressure in spite of blood loss. This sympathetic response to injury masks early signs of hypovolemic shock.

Δ Children can lose up to 25% of their circulating blood volume *before* a drop in their BP is seen.

Δ Children have immature thermoregulating systems that will complicate resuscitation efforts. Keep the naked child warmed with lights, heaters, and so on.

Δ Children have immature and pliable skeletons that do not protect internal structures.

Δ Children are still growing, so any untreated injury may result in progressive or permanent deformity and disability.

Δ Airway compromise, hemorrhage, shock, chest injuries, and central nervous system injury are the leading causes of death in pediatric trauma victims.

Assessment and Interventions

On notification of an incoming pediatric trauma victim, the ED team should prepare as in the *Multiple Trauma* guideline. However, special considerations exist for the pediatric patient, and the following modifications are essential in assessment and the interventions.

A. Perform primary survey and intervene immediately as necessary.
   1. Airway with cervical spine control:
      Δ position head in a neutral, midline position
      - flexion or hyperextension of the neck may compress the airway in an infant owing to the soft cartilage of the airway
   2. Breathing:
      Δ assess for:
      - grunting
      - head bobbing
      - stridor

- prolonged expirations
- nasal flaring
- retractions

Δ count respiratory rate for full 60 seconds in infants < 1 year old

Δ use blow-by O_2 when conscious children reject the oxygen mask

3. Circulation:

Δ insert two large bore IVs (18–20 gauge/children, 20–22 gauge/infants)

Δ consider intraosseous infusion for children 6 years or under, if IV not in place within 90 seconds

Δ send blood samples to lab:
- include type and screen or crossmatch
- perform bedside finger stick glucose test

Δ if child is in shock:
- administer 20 ml/kg bolus of warmed NS or LR over 5–10 min.
- reassess patient.
- repeat fluid bolus if tissue perfusion remains inadequate.
- reassess patient.
- if shock continues after two fluid boluses, consider 10 ml/kg of warm packed RBCs (type specific or O negative).
- if blood is not available, consider albumin.

 ALERT A child in hypovolemic shock often requires at least 40–60 mL/kg of fluid in the first hour of resuscitation.

4. Disability:

Δ assess mental status

A = **A**lert

V = **V**erbal response

P = **P**ain

U = **U**nresponsive

Δ assign pediatric trauma score (see charts following this guideline)

B. Perform secondary survey and intervene as necessary.

1. Expose and examine:

Δ briefly scan body

Δ undress patient

Δ initiate warming methods
- warmed oxygen
- warmed blankets
- radiant warmer

2. Vital signs:

Δ obtain respiratory rate, apical pulse, blood pressure

Δ obtain rectal temperature

3. History (in addition to subjective data from Multiple Trauma guideline):
   Δ immunization status
   Δ for infants, determine birth history
4. Head-to-toe assessment:
   Δ head, face, and neck
   • infant anterior and posterior fontanelles detect fullness or bulging
   • *Raccoon's eyes:* periorbital ecchymosis that may indicate a head injury 12–24 hours old and a possible basilar skull fracture
   • *Battle's sign:* ecchymosis over the mastoid area that may indicate an injury 12–24 hours old and possible basilar skull fracture
   Δ chest, clavicles
   Δ abdomen
   • may take 12–24 hours for intra-abdominal injuries to be obvious
   • insert orogastric or nasogastric tube to decompress stomach
   Δ posterior pelvis and genitalia
   Δ extremities
   Δ assessment (same procedure as with adults)
C. Document:
   Δ initial assessment
   Δ reassessments
   Δ interventions
   Δ serial vital signs

Pediatric Emergency Equipment

| Age and Weight | Airway/Breathing | | | | Circulation | Other | |
	Oxygen Mask	ET Tube	Bag-Valve Mask	Suction	BP Cuff	IV Catheter	Foley Catheter
Premie (1–1.5 kg)	Premie Newborn	2.5 Uncuffed	Infant	6–8 Fr	Premie Newborn	22, 24	5
0–6 months (3.5–7.5 kg)	Newborn	3.0 Uncuffed	Infant	8 FR	Newborn Infant	20, 22, 24	5
6–12 months (7.5–10 kg)	Pediatric	3.0 Uncuffed	Pediatric	8–10 Fr	Infant Child	20, 22, 24	5,8
1–3 years (10–15 kg)	Pediatric	3.5–4.5 Uncuffed	Pediatric	10 Fr	Child	16, 18, 20, 22	8, 10
4–7 years (17.5–23 kg)	Pediatric	5.0–6.0 Uncuffed	Pediatric	14 Fr	Child	16, 18, 20	10
>7 years (>24 kg)	Adult	6.0 Cuffed	Pediatric Adult	14 Fr	Child Adult	14, 16, 18	10

     Δ input/output

     Δ immunizations

     Δ injury inventory (consider using Pediatric Injury Assessment form)

  D. Transfer to pediatric trauma center:

     Δ If facility is not a pediatric trauma center, consideration for higher level of care should be discussed and appropriate transfer arrangements implemented immediately.

Pediatric Trauma Score

Δ The *pediatric trauma score* (PTS) is similar to the trauma score and the revised score.

  • Critical pediatric assessment areas are given special attention.

Δ A number is assigned to each finding.

  • The total score ranges from no injury (+ 12) to a fatal injury (−6).

Δ A patient with a PTS range from 0–8 has increased chances of mortality.

  • The child should be cared for in a pediatric trauma center as soon as possible.

Pediatric Trauma Score		
Physical Indicator	*Condition*	*Points*
Airway	Normal	+2
	Maintainable with oral or nasal airway	+1
	Intubated or tracheostomy	−1
Weight	>20 Kg (>40 lbs)	+2
	10–20 Kg (22–44 lbs)	+1
	<10 Kg (<22 lbs)	−1
BP/palpable pulse	>90 mmHg (+radial pulse)	+2
	50–90 mmHg (+femoral pulse)	+1
	<50 mmHg (no palpable pulse)	−1
Level of consciousness	Completely awake	+2
	Obtunded	+1
	Comatose	−1
Open wound	None	+2
	Minor	+1
	Major or penetrating	−1
Skeletal fractures	None	+2
	Closed fractures	+1
	Open/multiple fractures	−1

Mechanisms of Injury From Trauma: Infant (Birth to 1 Year)

Common Mechanisms of Injury

Δ Airway compromise
  - choking
  - strangulation
  - suffocation
  - foreign body ingestion

Δ Motor vehicle-related injuries
  - with or without the proper use and placement of car seats

Δ Falls
Δ Burns (scalds or flame)
Δ Drownings
Δ Poisonings
Δ Baby walkers
Δ Child abuse
  - shaken baby syndrome

Injury Pattern	Risk Factors	Associated Injuries
Head	Head large in proportion to body Poor head control owing to weak neck muscles Pliable body structures and vessels predispose infant to diffuse head injury	Skull fractures: abuse, falls Subdural hematoma: abuse Retinal hemorrhages: abuse, traumatic asphyxia Diffuse cerebral swelling: MVAs, abuse, falls High cervical fracture: MVAs

Chest	Tongue large in relation to oral cavity
	Narrow airway
	Obligate nose breather
	Short trachea
	Pliable rib cage
	Mobile mediastinal structures
	Absence of valves in superior and inferior vena cava
		Respiratory arrest:
		  airway compromise, foreign body ingestion, obstruction
		Pneumothorax:
		  MVAs, falls, abuse
		Pulmonary/cardiac contusion:
		  MVAs, falls

Abdomen	Pliable pelvic girdle does not protect internal organs
	Portion of bowel adheres to spine
	Organs easily crushed between bony structure and injury object
		Laceration, fracture, rupture of solid organs:
		  liver, spleen, kidney
		    MVAs, abuse, falls
		Hematoma, perforation of hollow organs:
		  esophagus, stomach, intestines
		    MVAs, abuse

(Adapted from Miller, 1996.)

Mechanisms of Injury from Trauma: Toddler and Preschooler (1–6 Years)

Common Mechanisms of Injury

Δ Motor vehicle-related injuries
- occupant
- pedestrian
- bicycle

Δ Burns
- scald and flame

Δ Choking

Δ Animal bites

Δ Drownings

Δ Ingestions

Δ Minor surface trauma

Δ Child Abuse

Δ Firearms (preschoolers)

Δ Falls

Δ Sledding

Injury Pattern	Risk Factors	Associated Injuries
Head	Thin, pliable bony structures predispose diffuse cerebral injuries	Diffuse cerebral swelling: MVAs, falls Subdural hematoma: abuse, falls Skull fractures: MVAs, falls, abuse, sledding
Chest	Short trachea Compliant chest wall Mobile mediastinal structures Major vessels lack valves and predispose to traumatic asphyxia	Pulmonary/cardiac contusions: MVAs, falls, sledding Pneumothorax: MVAs, falls, abuse Traumatic asphyxia: MVAs
Abdomen	Pliable pelvic girdle fails to protect internal organs Proportionately larger abdominal organs Ribs do not protect upper abdominal contents Organs are in close proximity to each other Portion of bowel adheres to spine	Laceration, fracture, hematoma to solid organs (liver, spleen, kidney): MVAs, falls, abuse Hematoma to hollow organs (esophagus, stomach, intestines): MVAs
Long bones	Epiphyseal plates do not ossify until puberty; may mask a fracture on x-ray Periosteum is stronger and allows bone to bend, leading to greenstick fractures	Long bone fractures: falls, MVAs, abuse, sports

(Adapted from Miller, 1996.)

Mechanisms of Injury from Trauma: School Age and Adolescent (7–17 Years)

Common Mechanisms of Injury

Δ Motor vehicle-related injuries
- occupant
- pedestrian

Δ Bicycle-related injuries

Δ Burns
- flames
- explosions

Δ Drowning

Δ Falls

Δ Sports-related injuries

Δ Suicide
- ingestion
- gunshot wounds
- hanging

Δ Minor trauma
- superficial lacerations

Δ Farm injuries

Δ Penetrating trauma
- stabbing
- gunshot wounds

Trauma	Associated Injuries

Motor vehicle accident	Head: cerebral swelling, epidural/subdural hematoma, skull fractures, c-spine injuries
	Chest: pulmonary/cardiac contusion, hemo/pneumonthorax rib fractures
	Abdomen:
	    Liver—fracture, laceration
	    Spleen—hematoma, laceration, rupture
	    Kidney—hematoma, contusion, hematuria
	    Pancreas—contusion
	Misc: surface trauma, bony fractures

Bicycle	Head: closed or open injuries Chest: pulmonary/cardiac contusion, pneumonthorax, rib fractures
Burns	Surface trauma, risk of multiple trauma exists
Drowning	Respiratory: acute respiratory distress syndrome (ARDS)
Falls	Head: cerebral swelling, epidural/subdural hematoma, skull fracture, c-spine injury Chest: pulmonary/cardiac contusion, hemo/pneumothorax Abdomen and misc: same as for motor vehicle accidents
Sports-related injuries	Head: c-spine injuries Chest: rib fractures, pulmonary/cardiac contusions Abdomen: same as MVA possibilities
Suicide	Head: c-spine injury from hanging Chest/abdomen: variety of injuries from penetrating trauma, falls, MVAs
Minor trauma	Surface trauma: lacerations, contusions
Penetrating trauma	Head/chest/abdomen: variety of injuries to internal organs
Assaults	Head/chest/abdomen: closed or open injuries, fractures, c-spine injury

(Adapted from Miller, 1996.)

SKIN AND SURFACE TRAUMA (LACERATIONS, ABRASIONS, PUNCTURES, BITES, AMPUTATIONS)

Assessment

A. Obtain and record triage assessment that includes:
1. Mechanism of injury
   Δ mass and size of the wounding object
   Δ velocity of the object and direction of impact
2. Time of injury
3. Blood loss
4. Pain
   Δ location
   Δ quality
5. Paresthesia, particularly distal to injury
6. Immediate care of injured area
B. Assess wound for and document:
1. Dimensions
   Δ size
   Δ shape
   Δ configuration
2. Presence of:
   Δ edema
   Δ drainage
   Δ deformity
   Δ foreign body
   Δ devitalized tissue
3. Bleeding:
   Δ oozing
   Δ controlled
   Δ pulsatile
4. Range of motion distal to injury
C. Palpate (utilizing universal precautions) for:
1. Pulses distal to injury
2. Foreign body
3. Underlying deformity
4. Normal sensation distal to injury
5. Lymphadenopathy proximal to injury
D. Remove *all rings* from all fingers of patients with hand, wrist, or forearm injuries.
E. Complete remainder of basic triage protocol, and document accurately.

Interventions

1. Control bleeding
2. Splint area if suspicion of bony injury exists, and order x-ray (if facility policy permits)
3. Obtain aerobic and anaerobic cultures from deep within the wound
4. Remove hair around wound:
   Δ clip with scissors
   Δ do not shave hair from around wound (increases the risk of infection)
   Δ *never* remove hair from the eyebrow
5. Cleanse wound
   Δ abrasions
   - must be cleansed thoroughly as skin layers may trap foreign particles, forming traumatic tattooing when the area heals
   - use a high-porosity sponge or soft surgical brush and a non-detergent cleansing solution for scrubbing
   Δ lacerations
   - usually cleansed utilizing high-pressure irrigation with normal saline
   Δ puncture wounds
   - cleansing technique varies depending on injury
   Δ bite wounds
   - cleanse with high-pressure irrigation with copious amounts of normal saline
   - prepare for possible debridement of wound when necessary
   - assess for risk of rabies; may consider blood work if wound is obviously infected
   Δ amputation
   - place amputated part in plastic bag, and place the bagged part in a container of ice
   - *do not* place amputated part directly on ice or in solution
   - provide wound care to stump
   - administer dT per emergency department protocol
6. Consider IV placement for antibiotic administration for:
   Δ puncture wounds
   Δ open fractures
   Δ bite wounds
   Δ amputations

Pearls of Triage Wisdom

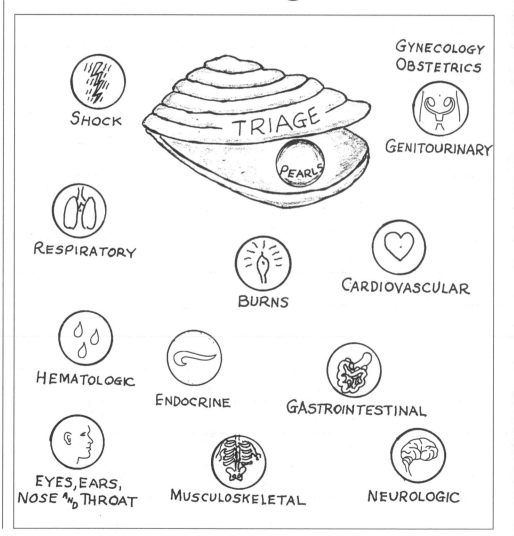

SHOCK

GYNECOLOGY
OBSTETRICS

TRIAGE

PEARLS

GENITOURINARY

RESPIRATORY

BURNS

CARDIOVASCULAR

HEMATOLOGIC

ENDOCRINE

GASTROINTESTINAL

EYES, EARS,
NOSE AND THROAT

MUSCULOSKELETAL

NEUROLOGIC

Notes

ASSESSMENT BY SYSTEMS

System	Assessment Finding	Could Indicate

Respiratory	• Stridor, inability to talk
	• Mental status changes
	  • apprehension
	  • anxiety
	  • agitation
	  • confusion
	  • restlessness
	  • lethargy
	• Severe chest pain, guarded posture
		• Airway obstruction
		• Hypoxemia
		
		• Chest trauma

Cardiovascular	• Changes in
	  • skin color and temperature
	  • decreased or absent pulses
	  • pain
	• Hypotension
	• Oliguria
	• Decreased LOC
	• Tachycardia
	• Tachypnea
		• Vascular compromise
		
		• Decreased cardiac output
		
		• Decreased cardiac output
		• Poor tissue perfusion
		• Acidosis

Neurologic	• Change in LOC • Bradycardia • Widened pulse pressure • Pupillary change • Paralysis or parenthesis	• First sign of neurological deterioration • Increased ICP • Increased ICP • Brain stem injury • Cranial nerve damage • Brain injury • Spinal cord injury
Gastrointestinal	• Vomiting • Abdominal distention • Tachycardia • Hypotension • Diaphoresis • Pallor • Pain • Guarding • Rigidity	• Bowel obstruction • Ulcer • Internal bleeding • Internal bleeding • Hypovolemia • Peritoneal irritation

Assessment by Systems (Continued)

System	Assessment Finding	Could Indicate
Musculoskeletal	• Deformity • Swelling • Decreased range of motion • Immobility • Bruising • Poor capillary refill • Pallor • Cool skin • Absent or diminished pulses • Paralysis • Numbness • Decreased sensation	• Fracture • Dislocation • Vascular compromise • Nerve injury
Eyes, Ears, Nose, and Throat	• Limited extraocular movements • Decreased sensation • Facial asymmetry • Hearing or vision loss • Local swelling • Redness • Drainage • Fever • Tenderness • Lesions • Nasal or neck swelling • Stridor • Dyspnea • Tachypnea	• Neuromuscular damage • Infection • Respiratory compromise

Endocrine	• Dry mucous membranes
	• Decreased skin turgor
	• Hypotension
	• Tachycardia
	
	• Alterations in LOC
	
	• Tachypnea
	
	• Bradypnea
	
	• Kussmaul's breathing
		• Dehydration
		• Hypovolemia
		• DKA
		• HHNC
		• Adrenal crisis
		• DKA
		• HHNC
		• Hypoglycemia
		• Hypermetabolism
		  • thyrotoxic crisis
		• Hypometabolism
		  • myxedema coma
		• DKA

Assessment by Systems (Continued)

System	Assessment Finding	Could Indicate
Hematologic	• Petechiae • Ecchymoses • Hematoma • Uncontrolled bleeding • Fever • Chills • Hypothermia • Signs of dehydration • Progressively decreasing LOC • Shortness of breath • Tachypnea • Cyanosis	• Coagulation disorder • Sepsis • Cerebral ischemia • Hypoxia caused by decreased RBCs
Gynecology and Obstetrics	• Tachycardia • Cool, clammy, pale skin • Restlessness • Fetal bradycardia • Fetal tachycardia • Hypertension • Edema of the face or hands • Proteinuria • Apprehension • Vertigo • Generalized edema • Tonic-clonic muscle reflexes • Convulsions • Coma	• Internal bleeding • Shock • Fetal distress • Preeclampsia • Eclampsia

Genitourinary	• Ecchymoses in the flank area
	• Severe colicky pain
	  • flank
	  • abdominal
	  • groin
		• Retroperitoneal bleed
		• Renal calculi

LOC = level of consciousness; ICP = intracranial pressure; DKA = diabetic ketoacidosis; HHNC = hyperosmolar hyperglycemic nonketotic coma.

▶ **GERIATRIC PATIENTS**

Δ The geriatric patient needs more time during triage, as communication with older patients can be difficult
  • The triage nurse must speak slowly and clearly.
Δ The triage nurse will need to determine how well the patient can hear, see, and speak.
Δ The triage nurse must continually assess not only the patient's physical and emotional condition, but also how well the patient understands the triage questions.
Δ When necessary, the triage nurse may need to rely on family or friends who are present to provide pertinent information.
Δ Many elderly tend to complain less often than people in other age groups do.
  • The triage nurse should carefully evaluate for the possibility of elder abuse.
Δ The geriatric patient frequently takes several medications.
  • The triage nurse should carefully document *all* medications the patient is currently taking.
  • The nurse may photocopy a written list if one is brought in by the patient, and attach it to the patient's chart.
Δ While assessing the patient, the triage nurse must remember that several factors influence the health of the geriatric patient.
  • Not all functional changes are related to disease.
  • Compensatory mechanisms decline with aging.
  • Injury/illness frequently occurs in "clusters."
  • There is increasing vulnerability to disease with aging.
Δ Aging also presents a challenge when considering drug absorption and distribution.
  • slower absorption of oral and parental drugs
  • slower absorption of drugs requiring acidic medium because of decreased acidity of gastrointestinal tract
  • slower absorption of suppositories because of decreased blood supply to the rectum and lower body temperature
  • slower drug distribution because of reduction of active and passive transport systems
  • greater amount of pharmacologically active drug present because fewer plasma proteins are available for binding
  • slower drug metabolism and longer duration of action resulting from decreased liver enzyme production caused by decreased circulation to the liver
  • increased concentration of drug resulting from decreased body mass and surface area and decreased renal function
Δ The following display lists the structural and functional changes resulting from aging.

Structural and Functional Changes Resulting From Aging

Body Systems	*Alteration*
Cardiovascular	Decreased distensibility of blood vessels
	Increased systolic blood pressure
	Increased systemic resistance
	Decreased cardiac output
	Slow response to stress
Pulmonary	Decreased strength of respiratory muscles
	Limited chest expansion
	Decreased number of functioning alveoli
	Decreased elastic recoil, small airway collapse
	Decreased resting oxygen tension
	Diminished protective mechanisms
Neurologic	Decreased number of functional neurons
	Decrease in nerve conduction velocity
	Short-term memory loss
	Reduction in cerebral blood flow
	Decreased visual acuity and speed of dark adaptation
	Decreased pupillary response and accommodation
	Increased auditory tone threshold
	Diminished sensation and touch acuity
Gastrointestinal/genitourinary	Decreased peristalsis
	Diminished acid secretion and thickened mucosa
	Decreased total nephron count
	Decreased glomerular filtration rate
	Diminished concentrating ability
Musculoskeletal/integumentary	Narrowing of intervertebral disks
	Bone density loss, increased risk for fractures
	Increased wear on joints
	Decreased number of muscle cells
	Loss of muscle strength
	Loss of skin thickness
Tissues	Decreased number of active cells
	Reduced tissue elasticity

(Andrews, J. F. [1990]. Trauma in the elderly. In *Contemporary Perspectives in Trauma Nursing*. Berryville, VA: Forum Medicum, Inc.)

▶ **MENTAL HEALTH PATIENTS**

Δ Triaging the psychiatric patient requires the nurse to be able to *sort through* the patient's medical and emotional needs.

Δ The nurse needs to remember the following.
  - Patients who present at the ED exhibiting aggressive and/or agitated behavior should be *considered violent until proven otherwise.*
  - *Never turn your back* on a patient displaying aggressive or agitated behavior.
    - Attempt to "talk them down" and seek additional help immediately.
  - *Be simple, direct, clear, and concise* when speaking to the patient.
  - *Remain calm* when dealing with an aggressive, agitated, hostile, or manic patient.
  - Be careful *not to overlook* other physical injuries or illnesses in the psychiatric patient.

PATIENTS WHO MAY BE POTENTIALLY VIOLENT INCLUDE THOSE WITH:

Δ history of substance abuse

Δ aggressive behavior

Δ verbal or physical threats of violence

Δ history of violent behavior

Δ history of childhood physical abuse

Δ suicidal or homicidal behavior

Δ presence of hallucinations or delusions

Δ presence of psychosis

Δ presence of organic, borderline, or antisocial personality disorder

Mental Status Exam	
Area	*Assessment Considerations*
Appearance	How does the patient look? Is the patient well groomed? How is the patient dressed?
Activity	Are there particular or unusual mannerisms? How is the patient's posture? What is the gait like? Is the patient agitated? Pacing?
Affect	A range of emotions *displayed* (happy, sad, unchanging, etc.) The patient may state he or she is happy, while appearing sad to others. Does the patient look angry, sad, depressed, elated or nervous? Are expressions appropriate to actions or words? Are expressions labile and do they change quickly? Is it difficult to determine whether the patient is feeling anything? Is the patient's affect flat or blunted?

Mental Status Exam (Continued)	
Eye Contact	Is the patient gazing with a fixed stare? Are the eyes darting about? Does the patient avoid eye contact with the triage nurse? Will the patient even open his eyes?
Mood	The prevailing emotion felt The *feeling* the patient states he or she has ("I feel sad.")
Speech	What is the rate of his or her speech? Slow? Fast? What is the volume of his or her speech? Is it clear? Is it slurred? Any strange speech patterns in how/what the patient is saying?
Thought Content	Topics of thinking and/or conversation Is the patient delusional? Is the patient hallucinating? Auditory? Visual? Olfactory? Tactile? What are the voices saying? Is the patient a threat to self or others?
Thought Process	Flow of conscious or mental activity as indicated by speech Are the patient's thoughts organized? Does the patient have a flight of ideas? Observe for rate, flow, associations, logical topics.
Orientation	Awareness of person, place, time, situation, relationships to other people

Memory	Does the patient have:
	    Immediate recall?
	    Recent memory?
	    Remote memory?

Insight	Is the patient aware of his or her own responsibilities and abilities? Is the patient able to analyze his or her area of concern objectively?
Judgment	Is the patient able to make appropriate decisions? Does the patient have good/fair/poor impulse control?

OBSTETRIC PATIENTS

Physiologic Changes of Pregnancy

Cardiovascular

Δ Displacement of the heart by the enlarged uterus will produce EKG changes.
  - left axis deviation of 15 degrees
  - flattened or inverted T waves in lead III
  - supraventricular ectopy may occur more easily

Δ Exaggerated splitting of the first heart sound, a loud, easily heard third sound.

Δ Systolic murmurs are common and usually disappear after delivery.

Δ Maternal resting heart rate may increase as much as 15 bpm.

Δ Tachycardia refers to a heart rate >100 bpm.

Δ BP remains at prepregnant baseline or drops 5–15 mmHg.

Δ Maternal blood plasma volume increases 40–45% over prepregnant baseline.

Δ Maternal blood plasma volume at term is above 4000 mL.

Δ Increased blood plasma volume without increased blood cell mass results in a physiologic dilutional anemia of pregnancy (Hgb 11–13 gm/dl).

Δ Owing to increased blood volume, clinical signs of shock won't appear until a woman has lost 35% of her total blood volume (~1400 mL).

- Special attention must therefore be given during a trauma situation, since the early signs of shock may be blunted.

Δ Peripheral venous pressure rises in the lower extremities because of the weight of the pregnant uterus, while remaining unchanged in the upper extremities.

Δ Central venous pressure rises from 1 to 5 to 10 mmHg in the third trimester.

Δ In the supine position, the large uterus compresses the inferior vena cava, and results in decreased venous return from the lower half of the body to the heart.

- This may cause arterial hypotension (supine hypotensive syndrome).
- Venous return increases when the woman turns onto her left side.

Δ Increased cutaneous blood flow dissipates excess heat caused by the increased metabolism rate of pregnancy.

Respiratory

Δ Increases occur in tidal volume (40–45%) and minute volume (40%).

Δ Respiratory rate increases as oxygen consumption increases.

Δ Increased total volume lowers blood P_{CO_2} causing mild respiratory alkalosis, which is compensated by lowering of the bicarbonate concentration.

Δ The base of the thoracic cage is shortened and widened, while the diaphragm is elevated to allow for the enlarging uterus.

Δ Increased mobility of the rib attachments allow the thoracic cage to expand.

Gastrointestinal

Δ Gums become hyperemic and softened, and may bleed easily.

Δ Heartburn easily occurs as a result of the stomach and intestines being displaced upward and laterally.

Δ Increased progesterone production by the placenta leads to decreased tone and motility of the GI tract that results in delayed gastric emptying and intestinal transit time.

Δ Hemorrhoids occur because of the increased venous pressure in the lower extremities and from constipation.

Δ Gallbladder may become distended as a result of decreased emptying time and the thickening of bile.

Δ Signs of peritoneal irritation are less reliable than in a nonpregnant woman.

Δ Abdominal rebound tenderness and rigidity are often diminished, delayed, or absent.

Urinary

Δ The ureters are compressed at the pelvic brim from the enlarging uterus, resulting in the dilatation and elongation of the ureters.

Δ Bladder is displaced superiorly and anteriorly, rendering it more susceptible to injury.

Δ Decreased serum creatinine (0.5 mg/dL) and BUN (10 mg/dL) occur later in pregnancy owing to increased renal blood flow and glomerular filtration rates (GFR).

Δ Glucosuria may occur as a result of the increased GFR without increased tubular resorptive capacity for filtered glucose.

Endocrine

Δ Slight enlargement of the pituitary gland.

Δ Moderate enlargement of the thyroid gland.
  • Basal metabolic rate increases up to 25% owing to metabolic activity of the fetus.
  • Increased thyroxin and protein-bound iodine levels owing to increased estrogen levels.

Δ Increased adrenal secretions and aldosterone.

Δ Alterations in the maternal insulin production and usage occur due to fetal glucose needs for growth.

Integumentary

Δ Increased levels of the melanocyte-stimulating hormone, beginning in the second month, produce changes in the woman's pigmentation.

Δ Striae gravidarum appear as reddish streaks on the abdomen, breasts, and thighs.

Δ Linea nigra is a dark brown line of pigmentation down the middle of the abdomen.

Δ Chloasma (mask of pregnancy) is seen as mottling of the cheeks and forehead.

Δ Angiomas (vascular spiders) may appear as small red elevations on the face, neck, upper chest, and arms.

Δ There is an increase in facial and body hair, a fine lanugo on the face and chest.

Δ Hair on the head may straighten, and an increase in hair loss may occur.

Musculoskeletal

Δ Hormonal changes increase the mobility of the sacroiliac, sacrococcygeal, and pelvic joints.

Δ The increased mobility of these joints may cause alteration in the woman's posture and lead to back pain and discomfort.

> ## PEDIATRIC PATIENTS

△ If a child is old enough to participate in meaningful verbal exchange with the triage nurse, *listen.*
  • Don't hesitate to ask the child about his or her symptoms.
  • The child must be made to feel important by the health care staff in order for a trusting relationship to develop.
△ Some children are good historians, some are not. Parents and guardians may provide the clarifying information when taking a pediatric history.
△ Be very patient when working with children.
  • Move swiftly if necessary, maintaining a calm manner.
  • Avoid conveying panic to the child and the parent.
△ Parents know their children better than anyone else!
  • If a parent presents at triage stating that "my child is not acting right," *listen* to their concerns.
  • This may be critical information that would be otherwise missed by the triage nurse.
△ When caring for a pediatric patient, the triage nurse should also "care" for the parent or guardian of that child.
  • If the parent is anxious, the child will be too.
  • If the parent is angry, issues regarding the child's health may become clouded.
  • Offer support and education whenever possible.
  • Offer concern and care to the parent and address issues as they arise.
  • Ask a reflective question to the parent directly, such as: "You seem upset, is there something you would like to talk about?" The nurse may find out vital information by this sort of question.
△ Allow children to make simple choices on their own, such as:
  • which arm to use for BP
  • what color band-aid to choose
  • whether to sit on parent's lap or in own chair
△ Parents or guardian may underestimate the seriousness of illness or injury in the pediatric patient (e.g., sepsis). Triage nurses must be keenly aware of the difference between parents' perceptions and sound nursing assessment of a patient presentation.
△ Nonaccidental trauma or child abuse should be suspected with any child when there are conflicting histories.
△ Obtain weights on all pediatric patients. For uncooperative preschoolers or toddlers, weigh the parent and child together, then weigh the parent alone and subtract to find the child's weight.
△ Count respiratory rate first, even before approaching or touching the small child. This assures an accurate respiratory rate. If the child is crying while counting the respiratory rate, document accordingly on the triage note (e.g., respiration 32/crying). By documenting the child's behavior, subsequent respiratory rates can be better interpreted.
△ Respiratory rates in children less than 1 year old must be counted for a full minute. Infants have a naturally irregular pattern of breathing and must therefore be evaluated for a full minute to accommodate for this irregularity.
△ Do all painful or invasive procedures last if possible. When painful procedures are done prior to simple ones, the child may distrust or fear all subsequent treatments and interactions.

Differences in the ABCs

Airway

△ Children have large tongues and their airway can be easily obstructed. Proper positioning may be all that is necessary to open the airway.

△ Airways have much smaller diameters and can be easily obstructed by small amounts of mucus or swelling.

△ The cartilage of the larynx is softer than adults, and the infant airway can be compressed if the neck is flexed or hyperextended.

Breathing

△ Sternum and ribs are cartilaginous and intercostal muscles are poorly developed, causing the infants' chest wall to move inward instead of outward during inspiration (retractions) when lung compliance is decreased.

△ Infants are obligate nose breathers for the first 6 months of life. Anything causing nasal obstruction can produce respiratory distress.

Circulation

△ Pediatric patients have a circulating blood volume that is larger per unit of body weight. Blood loss considered minor in an adult may lead to shock in a child. A decrease in fluid intake or increase in fluid loss can quickly lead to dehydration.

△ Tachycardia is a pediatric patient's most efficient method of increasing cardiac output and is the first sign of shock. Cardiac output decreases if heart rate is greater than 180 to 200 beats per minute.

Normal Vital Signs

Age Group	Respiratory Rate	Heart Rate	Systolic Blood Pressure	Weight	
				Kilogram	Pounds
Newborn	30–50	120–160	50–70	2–3	4.5–7
Infant (1–12 months)	20–30	80–140	70–100	4–10	9–22
Toddler (1–3 yrs)	20–30	80–130	80–110	10–14	22–31
Preschooler (3–5 yrs)	20–30	80–120	80–110	14–18	31–40
School age (6–12 yrs)	20–30	70–110	80–120	20–42	41–92
Adolescent (13+ yrs)	12–20	55–105	110–120	>50	>110

Remember:
• The patient's normal range should always be taken into consideration.
• Heart rate, BP, and respiratory rate are expected to increase during times of fever or stress.
• Respiratory rate on infants should be counted for a full 60 seconds.
• In a clinically decompensating child, the blood pressure will be the *last* to change. Just because your pediatric patient's BP is normal, don't assume that your patient is "stable."
• Bradycardia in children is an ominous sign, usually a result of hypoxia. Act quickly as this child is extremely critical.

Abnormal Vital Signs

Temperature: Hyperthermia

Δ Infants under 12 weeks of age with a fever of greater than 100.4°F rectally should be evaluated immediately.
  • They are less capable of localizing infections than older children.
  • These infants may harbor a serious bacterial infection while appearing benign.
Δ Bacterial infections must always be ruled out, including:
  • bacteremia
  • otitis media
  • meningitis
  • urinary tract infection
  • pneumonia
Δ The most common causes of elevated temperatures in children are:
  • viral illness
  • gastroenteritis
  • upper respiratory infection

Temperature: Hypothermia

Δ Infants have unstable temperature-regulating mechanisms, a high body surface area-to-weight ratio,
and quickly become hypothermic as a result of exposure.
Δ Hypothermia can lead to:
  • metabolic acidosis
  • bradycardia
  • decreased respiratory rate
  • cardiopulmonary arrest
Δ Sepsis and shock can lead to hypothermia
Δ *Every attempt should be made to keep all infants warm.*

Heart Rate: Tachycardia

Δ Common causes are:
  • fever
  • stress
  • anxiety
  • early shock
  • ingestion of a chemical substance

Heart Rate: Bradycardia

Δ *Bradycardia in children is always an emergency condition.*
  - Bradycardia may be signaling impending arrest.
  - Supplemental oxygen should always be provided.
  - Maintain ABCs.
Δ Other causes of bradycardia could be:
  - hypotension
  - acidosis
  - drug ingestion

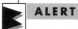 **ALERT** **Bradycardia equals hypoxia until proven otherwise.**

Respiratory: Tachypnea

Δ Common causes are:
  - fever
  - stress
  - poisoning
  - dehydration
  - respiratory distress
  - CHF (in children with congenital heart disease)
  - diabetes
  - ketoacidosis

Respiratory Rate: Bradypnea or Apnea

Δ Common causes are:
  - shock
  - acidosis
  - hypothermia
  - poisoning
  - respiratory failure

Blood Pressure: Hypertension

Δ Common causes are:
- increased intracranial pressure
- cardiovascular disease
- drug ingestion
- renal disease
- endocrine disorders

Blood Pressure: Hypotension

Δ Common causes are:
- shock (a late sign)
- drug ingestion

Beyond Triage

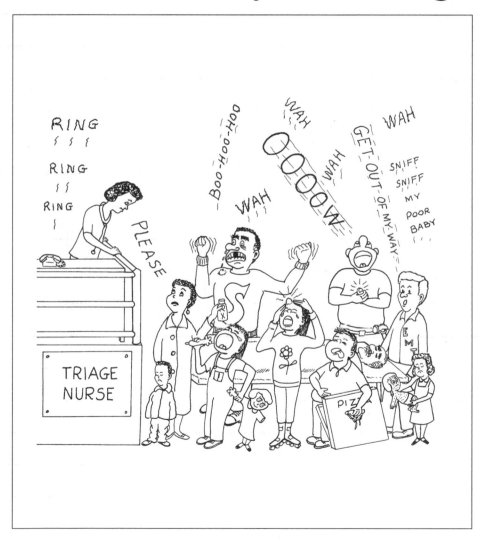

Notes

► CUSTOMER SERVICE

The professional health care staff must take a proactive role in offering high-quality customer service to patients, families, visitors, and colleagues. The excitement and challenge of the emergency department setting, which attract the attention of many health care professionals, also create difficulty in many of the interactions with those around us.

Chaos, crisis, noise, crowds, and high acuity are commonplace for Emergency Department professionals. For those other people who "visit" our department, those situations are sources of stress that add to the already difficult or unpleasant situation that brought them to the ED for service in the first place.

The nurse can create a positive environment by realizing that what may be normal for ED professionals is actually a great stressor for visitors. Whether it is a consulting physician in the department to see a patient or a family member worried about a loved one, it is the responsibility of the ED team member to welcome them into the department and express a sincere desire to facilitate their care and understanding.

Δ Start off your relationship with the customer in a warm, friendly manner. Unhappy or stressed people can often be cheered up or comforted by a simple smile. The patient carries more baggage than just a toothbrush packed in an overnight bag. Help your visitor to deal with difficulties, just as you would comfort your own grandmother during a difficult time in her life.

Δ Be personal with your guests and help to create a sense of warmth. Address your guests by name and be sure to introduce yourself. Your customers will feel comforted just knowing an ED team member by name, and feel protected if somebody seems to be watching over them.

Δ Offer assistance at every opportunity. By expressing a sincere desire to help, the ED nurse builds a bridge to the patient and his or her family. Once they understand that you are actively trying to help them, they will often cooperate more readily with whatever requests you make, and reward you with their gratitude.

Δ *Simple manners* on the part of the ED staff, such as saying *please* and *thank you,* outwardly illustrate your respect.

Δ Be honest and communicate frequently. Your patient and his or her family seek the same goals health professionals do and deserve to be a part of the process. Their stress level is already peaking, and lack of communication intensifies their situation.

Λ Always be proactive. When a person appears upset, angry or sad, take a deep breath, walk over to him or her, put a smile on your face, and acknowledge his or her feelings. The extra effort put forth and invested by the ED staff person initially often repays itself many times over in the long run. In some cases, your efforts may go unrewarded, but at least you will have the satisfaction of knowing that you tried your best.

No matter what your shift is like, there is always an opportunity to welcome those persons who are not members of your team and to teach them about who you are. You have the unique opportunity to provide everything from life-saving procedures to warm hospitality. ED professionals are members of a quality team, and this is an opportunity to show the world just how fine your team is.

CROSS-CULTURAL EMPATHY

The triage nurse encounters a large variety of patient presentations, some life-threatening and others relatively insignificant. All require professional expertise and care. When the triage nurse greets and assesses the persons requesting care, ethnic, religious, cultural, or social similarities are found between the patient and the nurse. Some qualities of each patient are similar to those of the triage nurse, and some differ. It is essential for the triage nurse to care for the patient and family without seeing differences as right or wrong, but simply different.

ALERT   The celebration of difference is the next step beyond mere tolerance or acceptance.

Culture is a broad term used to describe:

Δ intellectual development that has occurred with the evolution of familial generations of enlightenment, determination, and heritage
Δ style, beliefs, traditions, and knowledge passed from one generation to another
Δ the sum total of creativity, inspiration, and philosophy of a group of people within a similar belief system

Diversity is a term used to describe:

Δ recognition that people are different from one another
Δ different ways people engage in cultural practices that are different in origin or purpose
Δ understanding that we are free to celebrate differences without judgmental bias of right and wrong

As a health care professional, the nurse must understand that any differences that are not fully examined will influence the outcome of the health care delivered. In order for health promoting behaviors to be successfully developed, the relationship between the patient and nurse must be based on the acceptance that each person has the freedom to choose whether or not to behave in an established manner (McGregor & Barnet, 1998).

The health care professional is in a position to:

Δ Act as a culturally informed educator.
Δ Be sensitive to the fact that a patient's belief system may influence his or her acceptance and compliance with the prescribed or recommended health care.
Δ Act as a role model for others who are unfamiliar with such patient diversity.

The seasoned health care professional portrays confidence, friendliness, patience, and a gentle demeanor to assist the patient in coping with fear of the unknown and the uncertainties surrounding the ED visit. By offering a warm and welcoming feeling to *all* patients, the triage nurse increases patient satisfaction and compliance with prescribed health care services.

On the following pages are brief descriptions of diverse backgrounds, belief systems, and social circumstances patients live by on a day-to-day basis.

AFRICAN AMERICAN

Δ African Americans are one of the largest of many racial and ethnic groups in the United States.

Δ They had been one of the most focused on minorities until the 1990s, when affirmative action rulings began to emphasize all groups, minorities, and the disabled.

Δ Many families have a strong, extended family kinship.

Δ Grandmothers often play a strong role in the raising of grandchildren, especially when there is a single parent.

Δ Many African Americans are actively involved in church life, spanning numerous types of religions and belief systems.

AGNOSTIC

Δ This group neither believes in nor denies the existence of a God, as the evidence to prove or disprove God's existence is seen as incomplete.

AMISH

Δ This is an ethnoreligious group whose members live mostly in Ohio, Indiana, and Pennsylvania, as well as parts of the west and midwest.

Δ They are a conservative offshoot of the Mennonites.

Δ Most Amish are farmers, use no electricity, have no telephones and use manually powered farm equipment.

Δ Their central belief rejects worldliness and materialism; their style of dress is uniform and plain to avoid any pretext of vanity.

Δ Good mental and physical health are believed to be gifts from God, and hard work, a pure lifestyle, and a well-balanced diet contribute to good health.

Δ Worship is typically done at home, not in churches.

Δ They are stoic people and often refuse health care.

Δ Historically, they believe that immunizations are unnecessary, and death is regarded as the entrance to a better life.

Δ Most feel that life-support technology is inappropriate.

ATHEIST

Δ Atheists believe that faith in a *God* who directs human destiny, who hears and responds to prayer, and who loves and cares for his creation is unwarranted by either test of scientific evidence or rational analysis of human experience (Schmidt, 1988).

Δ The importance of each person's own credibility is stressed, as is reliance on individual knowledge to explain life events.

△ Atheists believe in neutral yet very powerful natural powers.

△ Atheists may be devoutly religious.

△ Patients may request the presence of others significant to them during crisis to provide human comfort and a sense of peace.

BAHA'I FAITH

△ This is an independent religion with 5.4 million followers worldwide.

△ Central teachings include oneness with God, religion, humankind.

△ Baha'is believe in harmony between religion and science.

△ When ill or injured, they will seek modern health care from providers they trust, and pray.

BUDDHIST

△ Buddha (c. 563–c. 483 BCE), who was known as the "Enlightened One," taught his followers how to achieve nirvana (inner peace) through morality, meditation, and wisdom. He taught that community peace could be attained through example, such as quality role models.

△ Buddhists believe that bad situations are often transitory and use their belief system to help overcome fear, anxiety, and apprehension.

△ Patients may believe that crisis is a result of a wrong committed in the present or a past life (karma). Many believe that if they are good, good will be done to them or a positive outcome will be their reward. Kindness from providers is a comfort.

△ Buddhism descends from Hinduism; many practices and concepts are shared by both communities.

CHRISTIAN SCIENCE

△ Christian Science was founded in 1862 by an invalid woman who was miraculously healed after hearing an inspirational speaker profess that disease was merely an error of the mind.

△ Believers seek to reinstate the original Christian message of salvation from all evil, sickness, disease, and sin.

△ Health is restored by the principal belief of divine harmony, and adherents choose spiritual healing rather than medical care. They may be aided with prayers for healing by Christian Science practitioners, identified individuals within the church who devote themselves to assisting believers with the process of spiritual healing through study of the Bible.

CUBAN-AMERICAN

△ Immigration to the United States began in 1959, when Fidel Castro took over the government of Cuba, and has not ceased since then. Early immigrants were well-educated professionals. That began to change in the 1980s with the Mariel boat lift. Cuban refugees then began to include dangerous and hard-core criminals, political prisoners, and those from the poor and less educated areas of Cuba.

△ Cuban Americans are spread throughout American society in both city environments and suburban areas around the country. Their inability to return to their homeland has made their cultural hold on their past weaker than others in Hispanic communities.

△ Cuban Americans have become active participants in American culture and tend to be active in politics, continuing education, entertainment, and sports.

FILIPINO-AMERICAN

△ Filipino Americans combine medical therapies with folk remedies. Disease is associated with total life situation and with both natural and supernatural causes. Spices are believed to have special healing powers.

GYPSIES

△ Diseases are divided into non-gypsy (*gaje*) diseases, which are treatable by Western practitioners, and gypsy diseases (*drabarni*), which must be treated by their own practitioners.

△ Disease is sometimes thought to be caused by the "evil eye."

△ Some foods thought to be lucky and necessary for good health are: pepper, salt, vinegar, garlic, and onions.

△ Family presence is vital to reduce fear and anxiety.

△ The "family" may comprise more than one "wife." The term "wife" refers to a relationship of duty or obligation. There may be several "wives," yet this is different than polygamy. For legal purposes, verify the family and patient's definition of "wife" before obtaining authorization for patient care.

HAITIANS

△ Haitians are immigrants from the mountainous island of Haiti, located in the Caribbean. Although the island is shared with the Dominican Republican, they have very little in common.

△ Most Haitians speak a Creole patois, a mixture of French, Spanish, and English.

△ The predominant cultural heritage retains its African roots. Santeria—a combination of Catholicism and African voodoo—is the primary religion. Haitians may use rituals of dance, music, magic, and cults of the dead for healing.

△ Amulets, charms, or herbs may be used or worn in prayer for preventing or curing evil or illness. Health care professionals should understand that removing these charms may create an emotional crisis for the patient and family; they should only be removed after careful consideration and discussion with the patient.

△ Haiti is the poorest country in the Western Hemisphere. Malnutrition among the rural poor is high, and malaria, tuberculosis, and hepatitis are common. Health care is difficult to obtain, with one physician for every 30,000 rural inhabitants (NewMedia, 1994).

HINDU

△ This common Indian religion evolved over several thousand years and intertwined history with the social system of India.

△ Hinduism has no founder, no prophets, no set creed to follow, and no particular institutional structure.

△ Hindu beliefs may be theistic* or nontheistic* and include: reincarnation, karma, natural moral law, and duty to follow within a divinely ordered society.

△ Domestic rituals occur for birth, puberty, marriage, and death.

△ Hindus number over 400 million worldwide.

Theistic: Traditions in which the holy is conceived of as a God, group of gods, or spirits personally involved in the life of human beings. *Nontheistic:* Traditions in which the holy is conceived of as an impersonal power, a process, a state of being, or an eternal truth capable of transforming human existence.

HISPANIC

Δ This term refers to persons with a native language of Spanish, a specific national origin, and a shared cultural background.

Δ Included in this group are: Mexican-Americans, Dominican Republic immigrants, Central and South American immigrants, Puerto Ricans, and Cubans.

HOMELESS

Δ Few social problems have increased as suddenly or been dramatized as effectively as the plight of the homeless during the 1980s and 1990s.

Δ At one time, the homeless person was invisible and ignored by mainstream Americans. Currently, the homeless can be seen anywhere and may include: "bag ladies" wandering the streets with their worldly possessions in a bag; men sleeping at the side of buildings, and runaway or throwaway children scrounging for food and shelter.

Δ The National Institute of Mental Health has estimated that one-third of the homeless are former mental patients who have been discharged under deinstitutionalization programs (NewMedia, 1994).

Δ Many homeless are addicted to drugs or alcohol, and common practice now includes the exchange of sex for drugs.

Δ Health issues among the homeless are staggering, and include: untreated chronic illnesses, rampant communicable diseases, and difficulty in finding affordable health care. Public health agencies find it difficult to keep up with this very transient population.

ISLAM

Δ Followers of Islam are known as Muslims or Moslems, and their beliefs embrace every aspect of life.

Δ This religion originated in Arabia during the 7th century through the prophet Muhammad. Common belief is that all individuals, societies, and governments should be submissive and obedient to the will of God (Allah).

Δ It is the world's third greatest monotheistic religion, with over 700 million followers.

Δ Islam emphasizes success, believing that it meets all of humankind's religious and spiritual needs.

Δ Daily prayer habits include praying five times a day while facing East.

Δ Dietary rules exclude the consumption of pork. Fasting is a part of certain holidays.

Δ Some patients may choose to pray before medical interventions.

Δ Because of extreme modesty, Muslims may request to have a health care provider of the same gender as the patient.

JEHOVAH'S WITNESSES

Δ This religion was organized in the United States in 1884. Their literal translation of the Bible differs from that of Protestants and Catholic churches.

Δ Witnesses believe Armageddon (the final struggle between the forces of righteousness and evil) and the second coming of Christ are near. Jehovah's Witnesses believe they will be the only ones to endure the Armageddon.

Δ Worldly involvement is avoided; Jehovah's Witnesses do not participate in nationalistic ceremonies and do not celebrate holidays by gift giving.

Δ No distinction is made made between clergy and laity, and patients may request that members of their religious group be present to comfort and talk with them.

Δ Most are *absolutely opposed* to blood transfusions.

JUDAISM

Δ There are varying degrees of religious orthodoxy and personal preferences regarding religious practices. Observance of the Sabbath (from sundown Friday through sundown Saturday) may be strict.

Δ Two key figures provide guidance, leadership, and education: the rabbi, the primary spiritual leader, and the hazzan, the artistic and spiritual role model who provides worshipers with the awe-inspiring chanting of the liturgy.

Δ Modern medicine is readily accepted. Comfort for illness is often found through eating (i.e., chicken soup). Some may follow strict traditional dietary laws. (Kosher meats tend to have a high sodium content.)

Δ Most are opposed to autopsy.

Δ Burial should take place within 24 hours of death whenever possible.

MORMONS (LATTER-DAY SAINTS)

Δ Mormonism was founded in 1830 in New York State.

Δ Sacred books include the *Book of Mormon,* and the *Doctrine and Covenants.*

Δ A common belief is that God was once a child, and that someday they may too, become gods.

Δ Bishops are considered spiritual leaders of the smallest unit of believers. They provide spiritual comfort during times of crisis, as well as advocate and arrange for the physical and social needs of the patient and family. The "laying on" of hands is used as part of their divine healing.

Δ Most do not use alcohol, illegal drugs, tobacco, or caffeine.

MENNONITE

Δ Mennonites evolved from Dutch and Swiss Anabaptists, who emphasized adherence to the word of the Scripture, strict church discipline, and the separation of church and state.

Δ The Anabaptists were the forerunners to both the modern-day Mennonites and the Baptist Church.

Δ Mennonites possess a deep concern for the individual's dignity and self-determination. Their belief system is similar to the Amish.

Δ Mennonites may accept modern medicine, immunization, and life-support techniques.

MEXICAN-AMERICAN

Δ Eighty-six percent of Mexican Americans reside in the Southwestern states, in search of a desirable style of living.

Δ This group of people is a product of historical development that began more than 4 centuries ago; they are the second oldest component of American history.

Δ In the past 50 years, they have emerged as a distinct and visible group. Most live in urban areas and share common problems with the rest of this country's urban poor.

Δ There has been an organizational movement since 1985; there are now more than 2100 Mexican-American elected officials in this country.

△ Strong importance is placed on family and extended family. Role obligations are seen as mandatory.
△ For those who have migrated to the United States without their extended family, the loss of that social, emotional, and economic support may be a major stressor during time of illness (Friedman, 1990).

MIGRANT WORKER

△ These are persons who move around in seasonal patterns looking for work.
△ Migrant labor arose largely as a response to industrialization.
△ As cities with their factory jobs expanded, people left farms for higher-paying work. The crops, however, still needed to be harvested. The lure of higher wages to people who saw no chance of improvement in their homelands pulled them northward into more prosperous surroundings.

MIEN (NON-CHRISTIAN)

△ *Sip mmien* ceremonies conducted by a male head of household or a Mien specialist may be performed to appease angry ancestral spirits. Such ceremonies may involve the sacrifice of a domestic animal, slaughtered by a packinghouse in a manner consistent with ceremonial requirements.
△ *Phat* is another ceremony whereby ancestral spirits are appeased in the treatment of ailments such as respiratory diseases or "soul fright." Cupping is a common practice.

NATIVE AMERICAN

△ This is a term used for the indigenous people of North America, covering a wide range of languages, habits, ethnic origins, and religions.
△ Migration for survival (hunting, cultivating) and competition with the expanding white population led to great dislocation, reaction, and interaction within the various groups and with Christianity.
△ Most Native-American religious systems recognize a cultural hero, employ themes from Christianity, and stress inherited traditional spirituality.

PENTECOSTAL

△ This is a modern-day Christian renewal movement that began in Kansas in 1901. This group practices a literal interpretation of the Bible, with informal worship services and enthusiastic participation by all.
△ There are over 22 million followers worldwide, and since the 1960s it has appeared within the established Protestant, Catholic, and Greek Orthodox churches.
△ Pentecostals believe in divine healing through prayer. Anointing with oil may be practiced with laying on of hands. Some believe illness is divine punishment, but most consider illness an intrusion of Satan.
△ Deliverance from sin and sickness is provided for by praying for divine intervention in health matters, and members seek to reach God in prayer for themselves and others when ill.
△ Most Pentecostals abstain from pork, alcohol, and tobacco.

PROTESTANT

△ This is a generic term used to describe the belief in the Christian faith that evolved from the Reformation as a protest against Roman Catholicism in 1515. The individual believer, not only the clergy, is seen as credible.
△ There are many denominations, including Adventist, Baptist, Episcopal, Lutheran, Methodist, and Presbyterian.

PUERTO RICANS

Δ As a result of the Spanish-American War, Puerto Ricans are U.S. citizens by birth. Many have settled in cities in the Northeast after leaving the island of Puerto Rico owing to poor economic conditions and high unemployment rates. There is a two-way migration pattern between the island and the mainland, and many find employment as seasonal workers along the East Coast and in the Midwest.

QUAKERS

Δ This is a Christian sect that was founded in 1667.

Δ This group believes that God is in every person and can therefore be approached directly.

Δ Religion is seen as a personal, inward experience.

Δ Simplicity is emphasized in all things; followers are active promoters of tolerance, justice, peace, and are often conscientious objectors during wartime. An example of their belief commitment occurred in the early 18th century, when they played a significant part in the abolition of slavery.

ROMAN CATHOLICS

Δ Believers of Christian doctrine, *the people of God.* Church doctrines have remained largely untouched since its beginning, and followers accept the traditions as authoritative.

Δ The Vatican (an independent state in Rome), under the direction of the Pope, implements policy and controls this vast and complex organization.

Δ Principal doctrines include: God as trinity, redemption, creation, the *place* of the Holy Spirit, and the *person* and the *work* of Jesus Christ (Wadsworth, 1995).

Δ It is important to understand that Catholics may believe that the souls of infants who die unbaptized will float through eternity. Any layperson may baptize an infant with a sprinkle of water, saying "I baptize you in the name of the Father, Son, and Holy Ghost."

Δ Some critically ill patients may request to have a priest called to administer the Sacrament of the Sick. Having access to a prayer book or rosary beads may bring comfort.

SEXUAL ORIENTATION

Δ Characteristics of human sexuality involve biological, psychological, and sociological behaviors. Sexual orientation is very complex and has been studied and included in every civilization throughout history.

Δ As individual's affiliation with a particular religious, social, ethnic, or cultural group may be influenced by the group's attitudes that may allow, encourage, or condemn a person's right to choose a sexual identity other than adult heterosexuality.

Δ A person's right to choose is monitored and lobbied for by numerous civil rights groups in the United States. Equal opportunity in employment, housing, business, and health care is sought and obtained. The courts become involved when issues of discrimination based on sexual orientation arise.

SOUTHEAST ASIANS (CHINESE, CAMBODIANS, INDOCHINESE)

Δ People who belong to this group may believe that illness is a result of weak nerves, imbalance of *yin* and *yang,* an obstruction of *chi* (life energy), disharmony with nature, a curse, or as a punishment for immorality.

Δ Coining, cupping, burning, pinching, and moxibustion may be practiced.

Δ Herbal remedies are commonly used.

Δ Trust and security rarely extend beyond the family.

Δ Most are sensitive to social class distinctions, and their modesty may require caregivers and translators of the same gender as the patient.

Δ They may speak at least one of the following: Vietnamese, Cambodian, Laotian, or Hmong (a Laotian tribal language).

Δ *Amulets* are simple black strings with several large knots, and are worn around the wrist, waist, or neck. They represent prayers for preventing or curing evil or illness. Health care professionals should understand that removing an amulet may create an emotional crisis for the patient and family. It should be removed only after careful consideration and discussion with the patient.

VIETNAMESE

Δ Immediate and extended families are very valuable. Mothers generally care for children for the first 2 years of life, after which paternal grandmothers assume much of the responsibility.

Δ Religions practiced include a combination of Buddhism, Confucianism, Taoism, and Roman Catholicism.

Δ Health concepts are heavily influenced by their religious beliefs, including: illness results from a bad deed in this or a previous life; a balance between *yin* and *yang* forces maintains immunity and prevents disease.

(FORMER) YUGOSLAVIA (BOSNIA, CROATIA, HERZEGOVINA, MACEDONIA, SERBIA, SLOVENIA)

Δ As a result of the civil war and political conflict in the former Yugoslavia, terrible tolls have been exacted on adults and children.

Δ Most health care resources have been focused on survival. Routine care of chronic illnesses, health maintenance, and care for the young has been nonexistent.

Δ Over 17,000 children have died since the beginning of the war.

Δ Persons surviving the war are experiencing an increase in devastating mental health illness; mortality for common health issues; complications of routine congenital defects, injuries, and chronic illnesses; and infant mortality and birth defects (National Research Council, 1994).

Common Cultural Practices

Practice	Treatment For	Process	Appearance
Burning	• Pain • Cough • Diarrhea • Failure to thrive	A dried weed is dipped in hot lard, ignited, and applied to the skin.	Asymmetric, superficial painful burns on the forehead, neck, front or back of the body
Coining/ Rubbing	• Fever • Pain • Colds • Vomiting • Headache • Muscle cramps	The edge of a smooth metallic coin or spoon is dipped in menthol oil and rubbed vigorously downward over the symptomatic area.	Superficial ecchymotic areas that typically occur in a striped pattern May appear as parallel linear marks on or near the spine, ribs, trachea, or upper arms
Cupping	• Fever • Headache • Cold • Cough • Dizziness • Pain	A heated cup is placed on the skin, where a vacuum forms. The cup is left in place for up to 30 minutes on the trunk, shoulder, or forehead.	Symmetrical flat, circular ecchymotic areas Appear on chest, abdomen, back or forehead May be painful to touch The number of areas produced can indicate the severity of the patient's symptoms and the length of the current illness.
Moxibustion	• Abdominal pain • Diarrhea • Ulcers • Hernia	The moxa herb or other incense is slowly smoldered near the skin.	Often resemble cigarette burns May be in a pyramid shape Appear on the abdomen, chest, or back
Pinching	• Headache • Cold or flu • Pain • Fever • Heat exhaustion • Fainting • Stomachache • Vomiting • Diarrhea	Skin is lubricated with metholated ointment and massaged before pinching occurs	Small welts or ecchymotic areas in a regular pattern May be seen in a pattern of two or three vertical rows on the neck, face, forehead, trachea, chest, upper arms, spine, or back
Sweeping (with an egg)	• Fever • Headache • Restlessness • Crying • Vomiting	Egg may be rolled on the body to pick up evil or demons and then used to transport them away. Egg may also be used in a ceremony near the patient's bed.	Often no visible signs of this treatment
Sweeping (using orange, lemon, or palm leaves)	• Anorexia • Fatigue • Insomnia • Hallucinations • Weakness	A healer (often a grandmother) uses branches or leaves to sweep over the patient's body while reciting prayers. An herbal tea may be administered after this procedure.	May not leave any physical marks on the patient May account for a delay in seeking modern health care

Beckman-Murray & Proctor-Zenter, 1993; ENPC, 1993; Handysides, 1996; Joyce, 1996.

HOW TO GET THE MOST BENEFIT FROM AN INTERPRETER

Communication is a key element in the health care professional's ability to work with, care for, and educate patients and their families.

When the patient is a non–English-speaking person, the communication process requires additional patience and concentration on the part of the professional. For communication to be successful, the ED staff must:

Δ Avoid lengthy conversations
Δ Utilize short, understandable phrases
Δ Use questions that elicit "yes" or "no" answers
Δ Be empathetic toward the heightened anxiety and needs of the patient

WHEN USING AN INTERPRETER, A FEW KEY POINTS SHOULD BE REMEMBERED

Δ Introduce yourself to the patient and to the interpreter. You may need to direct the interpreter to introduce you to the patient.

Δ Verify the interpreter's ability to translate appropriately. This can be done by simply stating to the translator, "I would like to see if my English is clear to you" and give some simple directions to follow. If the interpreter follows your directions and is able to communicate back to you, an assessment can be made as to the interpreter's ability to translate accurately.

Δ Let the interpreter know that his or her knowledge and assistance are appreciated.

Δ Face toward and speak directly to the patient. Refrain from turning to the interpreter and saying, "Ask her if this hurts."

Δ Be patient, take your time, and progress one sentence at a time.

Δ Resist the tendency to shout. Speak slowly and clearly; emphasize gestures, facial expressions, and tone of voice.

Δ Some patients may believe that it is culturally improper for children to know more than adults do and may not speak openly if a child interprets for them.

Δ Reproductive issues should be discussed utilizing interpreters of the same gender.

Δ Verify patient understanding of instructions by asking for return demonstrations or for the patient to repeat given instructions.

Δ By learning a few words of the patient's language, the ED staff member increases his or her rapport with the patient, as most patients appreciate the attempt made at communicating on a common ground.

Δ Document carefully if an interpreter was used and describe how the patient's understanding of medical care and discharge instructions was determined.

> ## BASIC SPANISH TRIAGE QUESTIONS

Δ Clear communication between health care staff and the patient is essential in the provision of quality care.

Δ This process of communicating becomes hindered when the patient speaks a different language from ED staff personnel.

Δ Optimally, the facility should have interpretation services available 24 hours per day.

Δ Times may arise when there is no interpreter readily available and communication with the patient must occur immediately to ensure the progression of quality patient care.

Δ Listed in the following are some common words and sentences to assist the ED staff in communicating with the Spanish-speaking patient.

Δ The terms are listed in English and Spanish, followed by the pronunciation.

In Spanish, the

G is like **h** before **e** or **i**
J is like **h**
H is always silent
a after a word is the feminine ending

Greetings

Hello / Hola (**oh**-*lah*)

Good morning / Buenos días (**bweh**-*nohs* **dee**-*ahs*)

Good afternoon / Buenas tardes (**bweh**-*nahs* **tahr**-*dehs*)

Good evening / Buenas noches (**bweh**-*nahs* **noh**-*chehs*)

How are you? / ¿Cómo está usted? (**koh**-*moh eh*-**stah** *oo*-**stehd**?)

Very well, thank you / Muy bien, gracias (*mwee-b′***yehn** **grah**-*s′*yahs)

You're welcome / De nada (*deh* **nah**-*dah*)

Yes / Sí (*see*)

No / No (*noh*)

Maybe / Tal vez (*tahl* **vehs**)

Do you speak English? / ¿Habla usted inglés (**ah**-*blah oo*-**stehd** *een*-**glehs**?)

I speak a little / Hablo un poquito (**ah**-*bloh oon* poh-**kee**-*toh*)

Greetings/Registration

Do you understand? / ¿Entiende usted (*ehn-t′***yehn**-*deh oo*-**stehd**.)
I don't understand. / No entiendo (*noh ehn-t′***yehn**-*doh*.)
Repeat, please. / Favor de repetir (*fah*-**bohr** *deh reh-peh*-**teer**.)
My name is . . . / Me llamo . . . (*meh* **yah**-*moh* . . .)

What is your name? / ¿Cómo se llama (**koh**-*moh seh* **yah**-*mah?*)

What is your address? / ¿Cuál es su dirección (*kwahl ehs soo dee-rek-s'***yohn?**) ¿Cuál es su domicilio (*koo-ahl ehs soo doh-meh-***sil**-*ee-oh?*)

Your telephone number? / ¿Su número de teléfono (*soo* **noo**-*meh-roh deh teh-***leh**-*foh-noh?*)

How old are you? / ¿Cuántos años tiene (**kwahn**-*tohs ah-n'yohs t'***yeh**-*neh?*)

What is your date of birth? / ¿Fecha de nacimiento (**Feh**-*chah deh nah-see-m'*-**ehn**-*toh?*)

Have you been here before? / ¿Ha estado aquí antes (*ah eh-***stah**-*doh ah-***kee** *ahn-tehs?*)

Where do you work? / ¿Dónde trabaja (**Dohn**-*deh trah-***bah**-*hah?*)

Please sign here. / Por favor, firme aquí (*Pohr fah-***bohr** *feer-meh ah-***kee.**)

You are giving us permission to treat you here. / Usted nos da permiso de tratarlo(a) aquí. (**Oos**-*tehd nohs* **dah** *pehr-***mee**-*soh deh trah-***tahr**-*loh[lah] ak-***kee.**)

Where do you come from? / ¿De dónde es (*deh* **don**-*deh es?*) ¿De qué pueblo es (*deh keh* **pweh**-*blow es?*)

Triage Questions

What happened to you? / ¿Qué le ocurrió (*keh-lay oh-koo-***rr'yoh?**)

When did it happen? / ¿Cuándo ocurrió (**kwah**-*doh oh-koo-***rr'yoh?**)

Has it happened to you before? / ¿Le ha ocurrido antes (*leh ah oh-koo-***rree**-*doh ahn-tehs?*)

Who is your doctor? / ¿Quién es su doctor/médico (*k'***yehn** *ehs soo dohk-***tohr/meh**-*dee-koh?*)

Where does it hurt? / ¿Dónde le duele (**dohn**-*deh leh* **dweh**-*leh?*)

What medicines do you take? / ¿Cuáles medicinas toma usted? (**kwahl**-*es meh-deh-***see**-*nahs* **toh**-*mah oo-***stehd?**)

When was your last normal period? / Cuándo tuvo su última menstruación normal? (**kwan**-*doh* **too**-*boh soo* **ool**-*tee-mah mehns-troo-ahs* '**yohn** *nohr-mahl?*)

When was your last tetanus shot? / ¿Cuándo fue la ultima vez que se le inyectó contra el tétano (**Kwahn**-*doh fweh lah* **ool**-*tee-mah vehs keh seh leh een-yehk-***toh kohn**-*trah ehl* **teh**-*tah-noh?*)

Did you lose consciousness? / ¿Perdió el conocimiento/ se desmayó (**Pehr**-*dee-oh ehl koh-noh-see-m'***yehn**-*toh / seh dehs-mah-***yoh?**)

For how long? / ¿Por cuánto tiempo? (*pohr* **kwahn**-*toh t'***yehm**-*poh?*)

Do you have allergies? / ¿Tiene alergias? (**T'yeh**-*eh-neh ah-***lehr**-*hee-ahs?*)

Are you allergic to . . . / ¿Tiene alergia contra . . . (**T'yeh**-*eh-neh ah-***lehr**-*hee-ah* **con**-*trah . . .?*)

    foods / comidas (*koh-***mee**-*dahs*)

    dust / polvo (**pohl**-*boh*)

    medicines / medicínas (*meh-dee-***see**-*nahs*)

Do you have . . . / Tiene usted . . . (**T'yeh**-*neh oo-***stehd** *. . . ?*)

    asthma? / asma? (**ahs**-*mah?*)

    abdominal pain? / dolor abdomínal? (*doh-***lohr** *ahb-doh-mee* **nahl?**)

    backache? / dolor de espalda? (*doh-***lohr** *deh ehs-***pahl**-*dah?*)

    chest pain? / dolor en el pecho? (*doh-***lohr** *en ehl* **peh**-*choh?*)

    constipation? / estreñimiento? (*esh-treh-n'yee-***m'yehn**-*toh?*)

convulsions? / convulsiones? (*kohn-bool-s'-ohn-ehs?*)

cough? / tos? (*tohs?*)

diabetes? / diabetes? (*dee-ah-**beh**-tehs?*)

diarrhea? / diarrea? (*dee-ah-**rreh**-ah?*)

difficulty breathing? / dificultad al respirar? (*dee-fee-kool-**tahd** ahl rehs-pee-**rahr?***)

ear pain? / dolor de oído? (*doh-**lohr** deh oh-**ee**-doh?*)

fever? / fiebre? (**f'yeh**-*breh?*)

headache? / dolor de cabeza? (*doh-**lohr** deh kah-**beh**-sah?*)

history of heart problems? / ¿Existe algún problema del corazón en su familia?
   (*ecks-**is**-teh al-**goon** proh-**bleh**-mah dehl koh-rah-**sohn** fa-**meel'**-yah?*)

high blood pressure? / presión alta de la sangre?
(*preh-**s'yohn** ahl-tah deh lah **sahn**-greh?*)

indigestion? / indigestión? (*een-dee-hehs-t'**yohn?***)

lung problems? / problemas en los pulmones?
   (*proh-**bleh**-mahs ehn lohs puhl-**moh**-nehs?*)

nausea? / nausea? (**now**-*oo-seh-ah?*)

neckache? / dolor de cuello? (*doh-**lohr** deh **kweh**-yoh?*)

pain? / dolor? (*doh-**lohr?***)

rash? / erupción de la piel? (*eh-roop-**s'yohn** de lah p'**yehl?***)

sore throat? / dolor de garganta? (*doh-**lohr** deh gahr-**gahn**-tah?*)

stomach ache? / dolor de estómago? (*doh-**lohr** deh ehs-**toh**-mah-goh?*)

vaginal discharge? / una secreción vaginal anormal?
   (**oo**-*nah seh-kreh-s'**yohn** vah-hee-**nahl** ah-nohr-**mahl?***)

vomiting? / vómitos? (**voh**-*mee-tos?*)

insurance? / ¿plan médico? (*plahn **meh**-dee-ko?*)

General Information

Are you pregnant? / Está embarazada? (*eh-**stah** ehm-bah-rah-**sah**-dah?*)

You will need an X-ray. / Necesita una radiografía. (*neh-seh-**see**-tah **oo**-nah rah-d'yoh-grah-**fee**-ah*)

You will need stitches. / Necesita puntos. (*neh-seh-**see**-tah **poon**-tohs.*)

Your arm/leg is broken. / Se ha fracturado el brazo/la pierna.
   (*seh ah frahk-too-**rah**-doh ehl **brah**-soh/lah p'**yehr**-nah.*)

It is only a sprain. / Es una torcedura solamente.
   (ehs **oo**-*nah tohr-seh-**doo**-rah soh-lah-**mehn**-teh.*)

I am calling a specialist to see you. / Voy a llamar a un especialista para que lo/la vea.
   (voy ah yah-**mahr** *ah oon eh-speh-s'*yah-**lee**-*stah pah-rah keh loh[lah]* **veh**-*ah.*)

You will need an operation. / Necesita una operación (cirugia).
   (*neh-seh-**see**-tah **oo**-nah oh-peh-rah-s'**yohn** [see-roo-**hee**-ah].*)

I am going to give you an injection. / Le voy a poner una inyección.

(*leh voy ah poh-***nehr** oo-*nah een-yehk-s'***yohn.**)

You will have to wait 30 minutes. / Tendrá que esperar por lo menos treinta minutos.

(*Tehn-***drah** *keh ehs-peh-***rahr** *pohr loh* **meh-***nohs* **train-***tah mee-***noo-***tohs.*)

I am going to place an intravenous needle in your arm. /

Le voy a poner una aguja intravenosa en el brazo.

(*le boy a poh-***nehr** oo-*nah ah-***goo-***hah een-trah-veh-***noh-***sah ehn ehl* **brah-***soh.*)

Have this prescription filled. /

Haga preparar esta receta. (**ah-***gah preh-pah-***rahr** *eh-stah reh-***seh-***tah.*)

Who should we call to come get you? /

A quién podemos llamar para que lo/la lleve a su casa?

(*ah k'***yehn-***an poh-***day-***mos yah-***mahr** *pah-rah kay lo* **yeh-***veh ah soo* **kah-***sah?*)

1	one / uno	(**oo-***noh*)
2	two / dos	(*dohs*)
3	three / tres	(*trehs*)
4	four / cuatro	(**koo-ah-***troh*)
5	five / cinco	(**seen-***koh*)
6	six / seis	(*seh-ees*)
7	seven / siete	(*see-***eh-***teh*)
8	eight / ocho	(**oh-***choh*)
9	nine / nueve	(*new-***eh-***veh*)
10	ten / diez	(*dee-***ehs*)
20	twenty / veinte	(**beh-***een-teh*)
30	thirty / treinta	(**treh-***een-tah*)
40	forty / cuarenta	(*koo-ah-***rehn-***tah*)
50	fifty / cincuenta	(*seen-***kwen-***tah*)
60	sixty / sesenta	(*seh-***sehn-***tah*)
70	seventy / setenta	(*seh-***tehn-***tah*)
80	eighty / ochenta	(*oh-***chehn-***tah*)
90	ninety / noventa	(*noh-***behn-***tah*)
100	one hundred / cien	(*see-***ehn*)

January / Enero	(*Eh-***neh-***roh*)
February / Febrero	(*Feh-***breh-***roh*)
March / Marzo	(**Mahr-***soh*)
April / Abril	(*Ah-***breel**)
May / Mayo	(**Mah-***yoh*)

June / Junio	(**Hoo**-*nee-oh*)
July / Julio	(**Hoo**-*lee-oh*)
August / Agosto	(*Ah*-**gohs**-*toh*)
September / Septiembre	(*Sehp-tee*-**ehm**-*breh*)
October / Octubre	(*Ohk*-**too**-*breh*)
November / Noviembre	(*Noh-bee*-**ehm**-*breh*)
December / Diciembre	(*Dee-see*-**ehm**-*breh*)

► TELEPHONE TRIAGE

Telephone triage has become an essential part of health care in our society and around the world. Emergency departments, urgent care centers, and physician's offices receive telephone inquires from a wide range of patients in the surrounding community and from distant places. For telephone triage to be practiced safely and effectively, an organized system must be in place. Without a developed program to follow, the practice of giving advice over a telephone is unsafe in every imaginable way.

The goal of telephone triage is similar to that of face-to-face triage—determining the level of care needed by the patient and assigning an acuity level. On the telephone, however, a strong knowledge background, clinical expertise, established protocols, excellent listening and communication skills, and a sense of intuition guide the nurse. The nurse no longer has the additional senses (touch, smell, and sight) to assist in the assessment process and must rely solely on what the caller says and does not say.

Protocols are similar to face-to-face triage protocols, and a sample is included. The nurse performs an assessment and recommends treatment and when it is necessary—the level of care at the safest interval (immediately vs. 24 hours from now).

Sample Protocol: Abdominal Pain

    A. Obtain and record telephone triage assessment that includes:
       1. Description of pain
          △ **P**rovoking factors (what makes it worse/better)
          △ **Q**uality of pain
          △ **R**egion/radiation
          △ **S**everity of pain
          △ **T**ime (onset, duration)
          △ **T**reatment (what has the patient already tried)
       2. Associated symptoms and behavior
          △ known trauma
          △ fever
          △ irritability
          △ poor appetite
          △ chest pain

    Δ difficulty walking
    Δ gravid history
    Δ penile discharge
    Δ LNMP
    Δ last bowel movement
    Δ nausea/vomiting/diarrhea
    Δ difficulty breathing
    Δ urinary symptoms
- frequency
- hematuria
- burning

    Δ vaginal discharge or unusual bleeding
    Δ change in activity level
    Δ possible ingestion of chemical, plants, meds, etc.

B. Risk factors that increase the acuity of abdominal pain include:
    Δ history of abdominal surgery
    Δ diabetes
    Δ chronic/congenital illness
    Δ irregular menses in sexually active female
    Δ history of abdominal injury

C. See immediately
Triage nurse should advise the use of an ambulance when the patient's current status is life-threatening, may deteriorate en route to hospital, or anxiety level is too high to safely drive patient to closest ED.
    Δ recent abdominal trauma
    Δ pain is localized to lower abdomen (either side) for more than 1 to 2 hours
    Δ inconsolable child or constant crying for more than 2 hours
    Δ marked change in activity level for more than 1 hour:
- refuses to walk
- painful to climb stairs
- lying with knees drawn up to chest
- walks bent over, holding abdomen

    Δ severe pain if patient or child jumps on one foot
    Δ rapidly increasing pain
    Δ pain in scrotum or testicle
    Δ grossly bloody bowel movements or jelly-like stools
    Δ vomiting blood or bile on more than one occasion
    Δ possibility of ingestion or poisoning (plant, chemical, medicine, foreign body)
    Δ unusually heavy vaginal bleeding or chance of pregnancy
    Δ patient sounds very sick or weak to the triage nurse

D. See within 12 to 24 hours if:
    Δ pain lasts longer than 24 hours
    Δ urinary symptoms are present (frequency, burning, hematuria, etc.)
    Δ severe nausea/vomiting/diarrhea with risk of dehydration

Δ fever over 101°F (38.3°C), cough, weakness, sore throat

Δ persistent nausea/vomiting/diarrhea unresponsive to home care

Δ vaginal or urethral discharge

Δ weight loss

E. Home care advice:

    Δ Encourage lying down and resting.

    Δ Have vomiting pan handy.

    Δ Suggest sitting on toilet and trying to pass a bowel movement.

    Δ Offer clear liquids only and slowly progress to a bland diet for 12 to 24 hours.

        • May use rehydrating fluid solution for infants and small children

    Δ Recommend taking medications that may cause stomach upset with food.

G. Call back if:

    Δ pain worsens, develops new symptoms or if symptoms change

    Δ severe pain present after 1 hour of rest

    Δ constant pain persisting for longer than 2 hours

    Δ intermittent pain for longer than 24 hours

    Δ pain worsens with heat or activity

    Δ urine, stool, emesis contains blood

    Δ fever

    Δ persistent vomiting or diarrhea

    Δ increased concern or anxiety (Briggs, 1997; Brown, 1994; Kitt et al., 1995; Schmitt, 1994; Simonsen, 1996)

PART V

Post Test

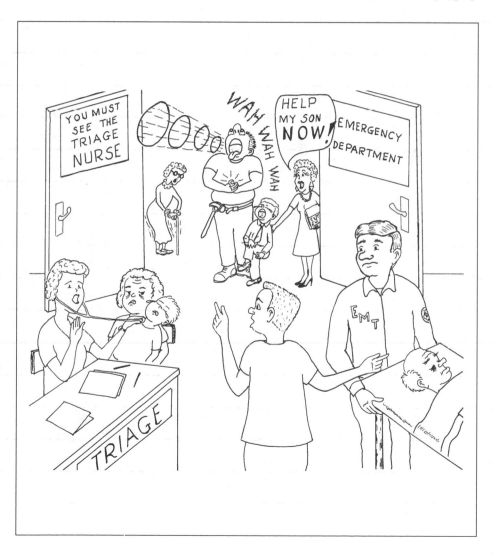

Notes

This post test is designed to:

△ **Acquaint the user with the quick reference style of this text.**
△ **Provide practice in utilizing the text.**
△ **Document a self-study or employer designated orientation or inservicing on triage with the aid of this text.**

1. Name three reasons triage is essential.

   1. _____

   2. _____

   3. _____

2. Which of the following is *not* a primary goal of an effective triage system?
   A. Rapid identification of emergent patients
   B. Assisting the patient in understanding the managed care program
   C. "Traffic control"
   D. Organization of patient flow

3. Name three advantages of triage.

   1. _____

   2. _____

   3. _____

4. A patient sensed a health care crisis in his or her life that necessitated a visit to the ED. It is the role of the triage nurse to assist this patient to regain _____ and increase his or her _____ of one's own integral part of health care.

5. The triage nurse's ability to recognize who is "sick" and who is "less sick" evolves through _____, _____, and _____.

6. Name four essential qualities of a triage nurse.

   1. _____

   2. _____

   3. _____

4. _____

7. Name four communication barriers a triage nurse must be able to handle.

1. _____

2. _____

3. _____

4. _____

8. The triage assessment, including documentation, should last no longer than_____minutes.

9. What is the responsibility of the triage nurse during times of triage overload?

10. What five senses are used by the nurse while triaging?

1. _____

2. _____

3. _____

4. _____

5. _____

11. Briefly describe what each letter in the mnemonic PQRSTT stands for.

P:

Q:

R:

S:

T:

T:

12. The triage nurse makes a triage:

A. decision

B. diagnosis

Each facility uses its own triage acuity system. For the purpose of this exercise, place each of the following patients in one of the three following categories.

Emergent/Life Threatening

Acute

Non-acute

13. A 19-year-old male construction worker presents with a chief complaint of crampy abdominal pain for the past 16 hours. The pain started in the periumbilical area and is now localized in the right lower quadrant. The patient has vomited once and has had no appetite. He denies diarrhea. He does not have a thermometer but admits to chills throughout the morning. The patient looks pale and uncomfortable.
    PMH: none. Medications: none. Allergies: Penicillin (rash).
    BP   110/76   Oral Temp   99.9   HR   96   RR   16

    Acuity Category:_____

14. A 56-year-old executive secretary presents to the triage desk complaining of burning abdominal pain. She points to her epigastric area with one finger and states that it has lasted for 3 days. The pain is present when she wakes up and when she is hungry. She denies radiation of pain. The pain is relieved with food or antacids. She seems nervous and somewhat uncomfortable. Her skin is pink, warm, and dry.
    PMH: none. Medication: Maalox. Allergies: none.
    BP   126/74   Oral Temp   97.8   HR   88   RR   16

    Acuity Category:_____

15. A 65-year-old presents complaining of a 36-hour history of mild, crampy, lower abdominal pain and a "full" sensation. The pain is worse with defecation. He has had one bowel movement is the past 3 days—he usually has one a day. He denies nausea, vomiting, or fever. His skin is warm, dry, and pink. The patient appears uncomfortable.
    PMH: mild hypertension, diet controlled. Allergies: none.
    Medications: Tylenol with codeine for a recent dental procedure.
    BP   152/90   Oral Temp   98.2   HR   80 and regular   RR   16

    Acuity Category:_____

16. A 26-year-old female presents complaining of feeling bloated and intermittent suprapubic cramping for the last 2 weeks. She missed her last period and believes she may be pregnant. Her last normal menstrual period was 7 weeks ago. She denies intense pain or vaginal bleeding. She is nauseated when she does not eat. She has no regular physician and would like a pregnancy test performed. She seems to be in no apparent distress.
    Medication: none. Allergies: none. PMH: none, with no prior pregnancies.
    BP   106/70   Oral Temp   97.2   HR   104   RR   16

    Acuity Category:_____

17. A 9-month-old infant is brought in by his mother. Mother states that the child has been cranky since yesterday and won't take his bottle. He awakes frequently from sleep, crying. The child is not wetting his diaper like normal and is not playful. The mother states his fever has been about 102°F; she admits to taking his temperature by feeling his forehead. The child is frequently crying during triage but comforts with Mom.
PMH: none. Medications: none. Allergies: none.
Immunizations are on schedule with private pediatrician.
RR 52 (crying) Apical HR 162 Rectal Temp 102.5 BP 96/p

Acuity Category:_____

18. A 2-year-old female is brought through the front door of the ED at 3 AM. The ED nurse at the desk hears a sharp, bark-like cough coming from the front lobby. The ED tech has already greeted the patient and would like to obtain vital signs on her before you begin your triage assessment. You see that the child is pale, awake but not playful, and seems to be drooling a little bit. As the triage nurse, would you allow the tech to care for the patient before you?_____

    Once in the exam room, the mother states that the child had been fine all day and went to bed very easily. The parents were awoken by this "horrible noise" and brought the child right to the ED. The child appears anxious and fearful. You ask the mother to undress the child, and you notice retractions.
Would you complete your assessment and obtain vital signs (before) or (after) you ask the physician to see the child? Circle One

Acuity Category:_____

19. A 3-year-old female is brought into the ED. The mother states that in spite of bathing her daughter numerous times, there is a peculiar odor about her. The triage nurse observes that the child seems to be well kept but also notices an unusual odor. The mother states that the child also seems to be coming down with a cold as she has had a runny nose for 2 days, but only the left nostril is draining. The child has no other signs, symptoms, or complaints.
Allergies: none. Immunizations on schedule with private MD. Meds: none.
HR 90 RR 24 Rectal Temp 99.8 BP 86/52

Acuity Category:_____

20. A mother comes running in the front door carrying her 5-year-old daughter, and the mother is screaming "Help me . . . help me!!!!" The triage nurse observes that the child is quite calm and is holding a paper towel around her thumb. The mother is very anxious and becoming angry that the child's care is *being held up* in triage. The nurse observes that there is a 1-cm laceration on the thumb, good sensation, capillary refill, and movement of the digit, and the bleeding is controlled. The mother continues to insist on immediate attention of a physician, and her voice is so loud that people in the waiting room are staring at you.
HR 84 RR 24 Oral Temp 97.1 BP 98/60

Acuity Category:_____

21. A 65-year-old man enters the front lobby complaining of chest pain. He states that the pain is a tight feeling in his chest and he has tingling down the left arm. The subjective assessment reveals that the pain began 1 hour ago while he was mowing his lawn. It was not relieved by sitting down. He denies shortness of breath, dizziness, or diaphoresis. He states he is slightly nauseated. The patient is pale, anxious, and has very dry skin.

PMH: noninsulin dependent diabetes mellitus. Medications: Tolinase 100 mg every day.

Allergies: none.

BP   148/90   Oral Temp   97.0   HR   92 reg   RR   20

Acuity category:_____

22. A 44-year-old women presents to the triage nurse stating she felt a sensation of pressure under her left breast 1 hour ago while she was walking her dog. She denies chest pain presently. Her subjective assessment reveals that the pain was relieved when she sat on the couch and rested. The pain lasted 20 minutes and was accompanied by mild shortness of breath. There is no dizziness or nausea. The patient appears slightly diaphoretic and in no respiratory distress.

PMH includes mild hypertension controlled with diet.

Medications: none. Allergies: none.

BP   152/94   Oral Temp   98.2   HR   84 reg   RR   18

Acuity Category:_____

23. A 17-year-old male presents to the ED stating that he needs a cardiac exam in order to play on the football team. He states that his last physical was 5 years ago, and he was told he had a Grade 1 murmur. He states that he does not have a regular physician. He denies chest pain, shortness of breath, dizziness, or syncope in the past or presently. The patient is a well-developed male in no apparent distress.

BP   106/62   Oral Temp   97.6   HR   58 reg   RR   14

Acuity Category:_____

24. A 48-year-old gardener is driven in by friends after sustaining a chain saw injury to his left arm 10 minutes ago. He complains of severe pain, and blood is dripping from a towel that is wrapped around the patient's wrist. There is a large laceration over the wrist with active bleeding, and the hand distal to the injury is pale and absent of capillary refill. The patient is unable to extend the digits and sensation is absent in the third and fourth digits. The patient appears pale, cool, and diaphoretic.

Medications: none. Allergies: none. Last dT: 8 years ago PMH: none.

BP   96/60   Oral Temp   92.2   HR   110   RR   18

Acuity Category:_____

25. An 8-year-old girl presents to the ED with her mother, complaining of pain and inability to move her left elbow. The child states that 30 minutes earlier she fell and tried to break her fall with her left arm. She denies any LOC or other pain. The child is tearful and anxious, bracing her left arm. The elbow has an obvious deformity with a large hematoma and swelling. The right radial pulse is strong, whereas the left radial

pulse is weak. Capillary refill on the affected limb is 2 seconds. There is normal range of motion in the left wrist and fingers, but the child is unable to move the left elbow. Distal sensation is diminished to light touch.

PMH: none. Medications: none. Immunizations are on schedule. Allergies: none.

BP   110/60   Oral Temp   98.8   HR   90   RR   24

Acuity Category:_____

26. A 17-year-old high school football player limps into triage describing right lower-extremity pain and inability to bear weight after a tackle during the game earlier that day. No other injury is reported. On physical assessment, the nurse finds point tenderness and mild swelling with ecchymosis along the middle portion of the right tibia. There is no obvious deformity and the foot is warm and pink. There are strong and equal dorsalis pedis and posterior tibial pulses. There is full range of motion of the right foot and knee. Sensation is intact to light touch at the medial and lateral surfaces of the foot. The parents of the patient have not been located and have therefore not learned of their son's injury yet.

PMH: none. Allergies: none. Medications: Ibuprofen 800 mg 2 hours ago.

BP   126/72   Oral Temp   97.4   HR   96   RR   16

Acuity Category:_____

27. A 36-year-old female limps into triage complaining of right ankle pain. She states that she twisted her ankle while walking downstairs in a pair of high-heeled shoes 12 hours prior to arrival in the ED. On physical assessment, there is a moderate amount of swelling and ecchymosis of the lateral right ankle. There is no obvious deformity. The dorsalis pedis and posterior tibial pulses are strong and equal bilaterally. Capillary refill, warmth, and sensation are normal. Range of motion of the right ankle is decreased owing to pain and swelling. There is pain on palpation of the base of the fifth metatarsal.

PMH: gallbladder surgery. Medications: APAP for pain. Allergies: none.

BP   148/98   Oral Temp   98.0   HR   104   RR   20

Acuity Category:_____

28. A 38-year-old man comes into triage complaining of severe abdominal pain and vomiting. The patient states that the pain has been diffuse since last night when he was drinking alcohol. He had two episodes of coffeeground emesis this morning, but denies blood in his stools. Patient appears pale, anxious, and slightly diaphoretic. There is a small amount of dried blood around his mouth.

PMH: consumes 3 to 4 beers/day. Medications: none. Allergies: none.

BP   100/60   Oral Temp   97.0   HR   120 and weak   RR   22

Acuity Category:_____

29. What should be done immediately with an aggressive, manic, or suicidal patient in triage?

30. Name six patient conditions that are considered high risk.

1. _____

2. _____

3. _____

4. _____

5. _____

6. _____

31. How soon after presentation should a patient with chest pain have an EKG performed?

32. Describe three signs a triage nurse must assess for a patient complaining of difficulty breathing.

1. _____

2. _____

3. _____

33. When would a urine sample be appropriate to obtain on a patient from triage?

34. When assessing a 9-month-old infant, for how long would you count a respiratory rate?

35. Name the five characteristics of headache pain that the triage nurse should assess.

1. _____

2. _____

3. _____

4. _____

5. _____

36. The triage nurse determines that a 62-year-old woman with a deformed wrist will be sent to x-ray after the triage assessment is complete. What should the nurse do before the patient is taken over to x-ray?
    A. Obtain an order for pain medicine.
    B. Remove the patient's rings and jewelry.
    C. Verify the patient's ability to pay for service.
    D. Administer tetanus immunization.
37. Withdrawal from alcohol can begin_____to_____hours since the patient's last consumption of alcohol.
38. Circle the correct word(s).
    If a patient presents with a penetrating injury to the eye, the triage nurse (should) (should not) remove the foreign body.
39. If a patient walks into the ED with a history of a possible cervical spine trauma, the triage nurse can assume that no injury has occurred because the patient is ambulatory.
    A. True
    B. False
40. The triage nurse should suspect child abuse in a toddler with third-degree burns on the hand that appear
    A. Splattered
    B. Asymmetric
    C. Nondemarcated
    D. Circumferential
41. The triage nurse might suspect child abuse or neglect in a 13-month-old boy who:
    A. Clings to his mother
    B. Moves away from the emergency nurse
    C. Avoids eye contact with his mother
    D. Sucks his thumb
42. The pediatric patient in hypovolemic shock should receive an initial IV bolus of warmed Normal Saline or Lactated Ringer's over 5 to 10 minutes. The calculated amount should be:
    A. 20 cc/Kg
    B. 30 cc/Kg
    C. 40 cc/Kg
    D. 50 cc/Kg
43. During the first hour of resuscitation, the pediatric patient in hypovolemic shock may require as much IV fluid as:
    A. 10 ml/Kg
    B. 20 ml/Kg
    C. 40–60 ml/Kg
    D. 200 ml/Kg
44. When establishing and maintaining adequate airway, breathing, and circulation for trauma victims, the emergency nurse should give equal priority to:
    A. Assessing the patient's neurologic status
    B. Identifying all injuries
    C. Maintaining cervical spine precautions
    D. Assessing vital signs

45. Prior to beginning the head-to-toe assessment during the secondary survey, it is essential to:
    A. Ask nonparticipating personnel to leave
    B. Determine the patient's name and allergy status
    C. Notify law enforcement authorities
    D. Remove the patient's clothing

46. Bradycardia is always an emergency in the pediatric patient. Children who are bradycardic are considered to be _____ until proven otherwise.

47. Name four factors that influence the health of the geriatric patient.

    1. _____

    2. _____

    3. _____

    4. _____

48. All of the following are components of the mental status exam *except* identifying the patient's:
    A. General appearance
    B. Affect and mood
    C. Perception and cognitive ability
    D. Organ system pathology

49. Women experiencing a spontaneous abortion (will) (will not) need support while coping with their loss.

50. Describe the difference between the Trauma Score and the Revised Trauma Score.
    _____

51. The term "Hispanic" means: _____

52. The cultural practice that appears as circular, nonraised ecchymotic areas on the skin is called:
    A. Coining
    B. Cupping
    C. Moxibustion
    D. Pinching

53. Which of the following statements best interprets these results of a visual acuity exam done on a patient? 20/40 −2 OD
    A. The patient standing 20 feet from a Snellen chart read what the normal eye can read at 40 feet, but missed two letters on the line with the right eye.
    B. The patient standing 40 feet from a Snellen chart read what can be read by the normal eye at 20 feet, but missed two letters on the line with the left eye.
    C. The patient read 20 of the 40 letters with the left eye and 18 of the 40 with the right eye.
    D. The patient read what a normal eye can read at 40 feet at 20 feet with the left eye and at 18 feet with the right eye.

54. When obtaining a peak expiratory flow measurement, the emergency nurse should instruct the patient to:
    A. Inspire slowly, then forcibly expire into the flowmeter
    B. Inspire quickly, then expire with slow, steady force into the flowmeter
    C. Take a maximum inspiration, then expire quickly and forcibly into the flowmeter
    D. Breathe normally into the flowmeter on both inspiration and expiration
55. Give an example of a skin lesion in which there is a necrotic hollowing of the epidermis and the dermis.
56. When utilizing the services of an interpreter, the nurse should face the patient during the conversation.
    A. True
    B. False
57. Which of the following means "where does it hurt" in Spanish?
    A. Que'ocurrio?
    B. Habla usted ingles?
    C. Donde le duele?
    D. Tiene usted asma?
58. All pediatric injuries should be evaluated for the possibility of:
59. Name four common mechanisms of injury in the toddler/preschooler age:

    1. _____

    2. _____

    3. _____

    4. _____
60. If your ED does not have an established telephone triage system in place, it is safe to give routine advice over the phone to patients not yet evaluated in the ED.
    True   False   (circle one)
61. Three high-risk factors for suicidal behavior are:

    1. _____

    2. _____

    3. _____
62. The clinical presentation of depression in the pediatric or adolescent patient is identical to that of an adult with depression. True   False   (circle one)

63. A serum glucose of what value would be cause to consider gestational diabetes in the 24th to 28th week of gestation?
    1. 100 mg/dl
    2. 125 mg/dl
    3. 175 mg/dl
64. Painful vaginal bleeding during pregnancy is a sign of:
65. Painless vaginal bleeding occurring between 28 and 32 weeks of gestation is a sign of:
66. If a vaginal exam is done on a patient with placenta previa, _____ may be the outcome.
67. When obtaining a history from a suspected domestic violence survivor, it (is) (is not) important to conduct the interview while alone with the patient.

Answer Key

1. 1. more patients seeking nonurgent care
   2. patients with no other doctors
   3. increased acuity
   4. increased violence in society
   5. illicit drug use
2. B
3. 1. patient is greeted by a registered nurse
   2. decrease in patient stress and anxiety
   3. assess patient before discussion occurs re: ability to pay
   4. emergent care expedited
   5. immediate assessment and documentation
   6. continuous reassessment of patient
4. control, understanding
5. experience, clinical judgment, and training
6. 6 months' ED experience, ACLS, PALS, ENPC, TNCC, certification in emergency nursing, precision skills in assessment, intradepartmental policy, supervisory and delegation, EMS knowledge, telephone triage, interpersonal communication, acting as a role model, decision-making skills, and problem solving
7. non–English speaking, expressive aphasia, intoxication, belligerent behavior, hearing or sight impaired, mentally handicapped, hysterical, or unstable mental state
8. less than 5 minutes
9. gain triage assistance from another RN, a supervisor, or a technician with obtaining vital signs
10. sight, smell, listening, touch, intuition
11. **P:** provoking factors
    Q: quality of pain
    R: region/radiation
    S: severity of pain
    T: time
    T: treatment
12. decision

Some of the following scenarios may fall into two different categories. The differences will depend on the "total picture" the triage nurse sees when evaluating the patient. For the purpose of this learning exercise, there may not be an absolute "right" or "wrong" answer.

13. acute
14. acute
15. nonacute/acute
16. nonacute/acute
17. acute or emergent
18. no, after, emergent
19. nonacute
20. nonacute (due to mother's increased anxiety, mom should have immediate attention to answer her questions and relieve her anxiety)
21. emergent
22. emergent
23. nonacute
24. emergent
25. emergent
26. acute
27. nonacute
28. acute or emergent
29. remove patient to a quiet room, arrange for one-to-one supervision, perform a suicidal risk assessment
30. refer to High Risk Triage guideline
31. immediately, within 5 minutes of arrival
32. tachypnea, tachycardia, bradycardia, room air oximetry, pallor, stridor, wheezing, cyanosis, retractions, crackles, ashen skin, nasal flaring, grunting
33. females with urinary complaints or abdominal pain
34. 1 full minute
35. onset, duration, character, intensity, location
36. B
37. 6–8 hours

38. should not
39. B
40. D
41. C
42. A
43. C
44. C
45. D
46. hypoxic
47. 1. not all functional changes are related to disease
    2. compensatory mechanisms decline with age
    3. injury and illness frequently occur in "clusters"
    4. increased vulnerability to disease with aging
48. D
49. will
50. 1. allows more weight to be given to the GCS
    2. more accurate assessment of the patient with an isolated head injury
51. Persons with a native language of Spanish, a specific country of origin, and cultural background; includes Mexican Americans, Dominican Republican immigrants, Cubans, Puerto Ricans, Central and South Americans

52. B
53. A
54. C
55. ulcer
56. A
57. C
58. child abuse or neglect
59. MVA (passenger, pedestrian, bicycle), burns, choking, animal bite, drownings, ingestions, minor surface trauma, child abuse, firearms, falls, sledding
60. False
61. adolescent, male, Caucasian, socially isolated, depression, hallucinations, delusions, intoxicated, lack of support system, chronically or terminally ill, prior suicide attempt, high-risk profession (refer to Mental Health: suicide information for complete listing)
62. false
63. 2
64. abruptio placentae
65. placenta previa
66. fetal hemorrhage
67. is

Glossary

A

Abruptio Placentae — Premature separation of a normal placenta from the uterine wall during the third trimester of pregnancy, resulting in massive hormorrhage.

Addiction — Loss of personal control with regard to a chemical or substance.

Affect — Moment-to-moment display or expression of human feeling.

Aggression — Any verbal, nonverbal, actual or attempted personal abuse directed toward another person or object.

Agoraphobia — Fear and avoidance of being alone, in open spaces, or in an environment from which escape might be difficult. Often presents as a fear of leaving one's own home.

Akathisia — Condition marked by motor restlessness and anxiety.

Alzheimer's Disease — Cognitive impairment disorder with progressive deterioration of function.

Anhedonia — Inability to experience pleasure.

Anorexia Nervosa — Preoccupation with food and eating combined with intense desire to control food, eating habits, and subsequent body image.

Aphasia — Difficulty forming words.

Apraxia — Loss of purposeful motor control and movement.

Autism — Condition in which thoughts are derived from an internal source with impaired social interactions and development.

B

Battle's Sign — Contusion on the mastoid process of either ear; an indication of a basilar skull fracture.

Bipolar Disorder — Mood disorder with variation between manic and depressive episodes.

Borderline Personality Disorder — Personality disorder involving impulsive and unpredictable behavior, especially in the areas of behavior, mood, relationships, and self-image.

C

Chemical Abuse — Regularly indiscriminate use of a chemical in excess quantities to the extent that a person's psychological, physiologic, and social functioning is impaired.

Chemical Dependency — Condition in which the body becomes so accustomed to a drug that body functioning is impaired without it; abruptly stopping the drug causes withdrawal signs and symptoms.

Compound Fracture — Opening in the skin over the area of a bone fracture; bone may or may not protrude through the skin.

Conversion — Unconscious transfer of anxiety to a physical symptom that has no organic cause.

Crisis — A person's reactive state to a life stressor.

D

Delirium — Disturbance in consciousness, accompanied by cognitive changes. Difficulty in mentally focusing, memory, language, orientation, and so on.

Delusion — Fixed false belief even when evidence is presented to the contrary.

Dementia — Insidious and chronic loss of intellectual function.

Depression — Refers to a symptom, a syndrome, a disorder, or an illness that may include overwhelming hopelessness and helplessness that are extremely painful and may be debilitating.

Drug Holiday — A brief period of time in which a therapeutic psychiatric medication will be discontinued or tapered to a lower dose. This allows the provider to evaluate the patient's baseline behavior and the possibility of maintaining the patient on a lower dose of medication.

Dystonia — Usually a side effect of antipsychotic medications, causing muscle spasms of the head, face, neck, and back.

Dysmenorrhea — Painful menstruation.

Dyspareunia — Painful intercourse.

Dysuria — Painful or difficult urination.

E

Euphoria — Abnormally exaggerated sense of well-being.

Extrapyramidal Side Effects — Abnormal involuntary muscle movements as a result of psychotropic medications. Dystonia, akathisia, and pseudoparkinsonism are reversible; the most serious, tardive dyskinesia, is irreversible.

Estimated Date of Confinement (EDC) — The estimated date of delivery for a pregnant woman.

F

Flat Affect — Absence of facial expression in response to emotion.

Flight of Ideas — Rapid movement from one topic of conversation to another—often difficult or impossible for the listener to keep up with.

G

Grandiosity — Exaggerated belief in one's own importance.

H

Hallucination — An alteration in the perception of a body sense when there are no external stimuli present (i.e., smell, vision, touch, hearing, taste).

Hypomania — An elevated mood in which the person maintains connection with reality and experiences no impairment of social, personal, or occupational functioning.

I

Ideas of Reference — Unusual or false impressions that outside or external events have a particular personal meaning.

Illusion — The misinterpretation of external stimuli (e.g., branches blowing against a roof interpreted as people walking on the roof).

Impulse Disorder — Abrupt and unplanned actions performed in pursuit of instant gratification.

L

Labile — Exhibiting rapid changes in emotion.

Looseness of Association — Illogical and haphazard thought process.

M

Mania — Extreme mental state of mood elevation with delusions, impaired judgment, and impaired reality orientation.

Manic Depression — Disorder of marked alternations in mood.

Melancholia — Extreme sadness that inhibits mental and physical activity.

Mood — Prevailing emotional tone (e.g., "I feel sad").

N

Narcissism — Intense self-love and self-interest. Normal in children; pathologic in adults when experienced to the same degree as children.

Neologism — Self-created words that have meaning only to the person using them.

O

Obsession — Preoccupation with persistent, intrusive thoughts that cannot be eliminated by reasoning.

P

Paranoia — Strong, irrational opinion unaffected by reality.

Phobia — Strong, irrational fear of an object, activity, or situation.

S

Somatization — The expression of psychological stress through physical symptoms.

Suppression — Conscious delaying of emotional awareness of a difficult situation or feeling.

T

Tardive Dyskinesia — Serious and irreversible side effect of psychotropic medications that involves involuntary muscle movements of the tongue, fingers, toes, neck, trunk, or pelvis.

W

Word Salad — A mixture of words meaningless to the speaker and listener.

Bibliography

American Academy of Pediatrics/American College of Emergency Physicians. (1990). *Advanced pediatric life support.* Dallas: Author.

Aehlert, B. (1994). *PALS: Pediatric advanced life support study guide.* St. Louis: Mosby-Year Book.

American Burn Association (1990). Hospital and prehospital resources for optimal care of patients with burn injury: Guidelines for development and operation of burn centers. *Journal of Burn Care Rehabilitation, 11* (2), 98–104.

American College of Emergency Physicians (1992). *Emergency medicine: A comprehensive study guide.* New York: McGraw-Hill.

American Psychiatric Association (1994). *Diagnostic and statistical manual of mental disorders* (4th ed.). Washington, DC: Author.

Anderson, R., Kochanek, K., & Murphy, S. (1997). Advance report of final mortality statistics, 1995. *Monthly Vital Statistics Report, 45* (11).

Andrea, J., & Renner, P. (1985). Interpreting needs of the ED patient: One California hospital's 3-week study. *Journal of Emergency Nursing, 21* (6), 510–512.

Andrews, J.F. (1990). Trauma in the elderly. In *Contemporary Perspectives in Trauma Nursing.* Berryville, VA: Forum Medicum, Inc.

Andrews, M., & Boyle, J. (1995). *Transcultural concepts in nursing care.* (2nd ed.). Philadelphia: J.B. Lippincott.

Beckmann-Murray, R., & Proctor-Zenter, J. (1993). *Nursing assessment and health promotion: Strategies through the life span* (5th ed.). East Norwalk, CT: Appleton & Lange.

Benenson, A. (1995). *Control of communicable diseases manual* (16th ed.). Washington, DC: American Public Health Association.

Boyle, J., & Andrews, M. (1989). *Transcultural concepts in nursing care.* Glenview, IL: Scott, Foresman.

Brewer, J., & Bonalumi, N. (1995). Cultural diversity in the Emergency Department: Health care beliefs and practices among the Pennsylvania Amish. *Journal of Emergency Nursing, 21* (6), 494–497.

Briggs, J. (1997). *Telephone triage protocols for nurses.* Philadelphia: J.B. Lippincott-Raven.

Brown, J. (1994). *Pediatric telephone medicine: Principles, triage, and advice* (2nd ed.). Philadelphia: J.B. Lippincott.

Cadwell, V. (1995). Christian Science and emergency care: A case of reconciling conflicting beliefs. *Journal of Emergency Nursing, 21* (6), 489–490.

Campbell, R. (1994). *American psychiatric glossary* (7th ed.). Washington, DC: American Psychiatric Press.

Centers for Disease Control (1998). *Morbidity and Mortality Weekly Report, 47* (8), 161–166.

Cergol, S. (1997). A different reality: Children and mental illness. *Genesee Valley Parents Magazine, 10,* 11–16.

Clemen-Stone, S., Eigsti, D., & McGuire, S. (1995). *Comprehensive community health nursing: Family, aggregate, and community practice* (4th ed.). St. Louis: Mosby-Year Book.

Compton's interactive encyclopedia (1994). Springfield, MA: Compton's NewMedia, Inc.

Cramer, C., & Cramer, A. (1995). Caring for the Latter-day Saint patient. *Journal of Emergency Nursing, 21* (6), 503–504.

Cross, L., O'Hara, M., Page, N., Robson, L., & Tompkins, J. (1988). *ABC's of pediatric nursing: A reference guide.* Syracuse, NY: SUNY/Health Science Center.

Denny, F., & Taylor, R. (1985). *The Holy Book in comparative perspective.* Columbia, SC: University of South Carolina Press.

Diseases (1992). Springhouse, PA: Springhouse.

Dubin, W.R., & Weiss, K.J. (1989). *Handbook of psychiatric emergencies.* Springhouse, PA: Springhouse.

Edwards, F. (1996). Dermatologic ED presentations: From the mundane to the life-threatening. *Emergency Medicine Reports, 17* (17), 173–179.

Eliopoulos, C. (1993). *Gerontological nursing* (3rd ed.). Philadelphia: J.B. Lippincott.

Emergency Nurses Association (1993). *Emergency nursing pediatric course: Provider manual.* Park Ridge, IL: Author.

Emergency Nurses Association (1997). *Triage: Meeting the challenge.* Park Ridge, IL: Author.

Epifanio, P., Manton, A., Carlson, K., & Marett, B. (1992). *CEN review manual*. Park Ridge, IL: Award Printing Corporation.

First rate customer service. #101 & #207. Fairfield, NJ: Economic Press.

Fleisher, G., & Ludwig, S. (1993). *Textbook of pediatric emergency medicine*. (3rd ed.). Baltimore: Williams & Wilkins.

Friedman, M. (1990). Transcultural family nursing: Application to Latino and Black families. *Journal of Pediatric Nursing, 5* (303), 214–222.

Frew, S. (1996). *COBRA 1996 update*. Conference at Niagara Falls Medical Center, Niagara Falls, NY.

Grimes, J., & Burns, E. (1992). *Health assessment in nursing practice*. Boston: Jones & Barlett Publishers.

Hafen, B.Q., & Karen, K.J. (1989). *Prehospital emergency care and crisis intervention* (3rd ed.). Englewood, CO: Morton.

Handysides, G. (1996). *Triage in emergency nursing*. St. Louis: Mosby.

Hay, W., Groothuis, J., Hayward, A., & Levin, M. (1997). *Current pediatric diagnosis and treatment* (13th ed.). Stamford, CT: Appleton & Lange.

Henderson, G., & Primeaux, M. (1981). *Transcultural health care*. Menlo Park, CA: Addison-Wesley.

Impact of war on child health in the countries of former Yugoslavia (March 1994). Workshop sponsored by Institute of Medicine and The National Research Council, Trieste, Italy.

Johnson, B.S. (1997). *Adaptation and growth: Psychiatric–mental health nursing* (4th ed.). Philadelphia: Lippincott-Raven.

Joyce, E., & Villanueva, M. (1996). *Say it in Spanish*. Philadelphia: W.B. Saunders.

Kaminester, L. (1991). *Sexually transmitted diseases: An illustrated guide to differential diagnosis*. Triangle Park, NC: Burroughs Wellcome.

Kidd, P.S., & Murakami, R. (1987). Common pathologic conditions in elderly person: Nursing assessment and interventions. *Journal of Emergency Nursing, 13* (1), 31.

Kirksey, K., et al. (1995). Thoughts on care for transsexual patients. *Journal of Emergency Nursing, 21* (6), 519–520.

Kitt, S., Selfridge-Thomas, J., Proehl, J., & Kaiser, J. (1995). *Emergency nursing: A physiologic and clinical perspective* (2nd ed.). Philadelphia: W.B. Saunders.

Klein, A., Lee, G., Manton, A., & Parker, J. (1994). *Emergency nursing core curriculum* (4th ed.). Philadelphia: W.B. Saunders.

Langley, M. (1981). *A book of beliefs: Religions*. Ontario, Canada: Paideia Press.

Lippincott manual of nursing practice (5th ed.). (1991). Philadelphia: J.B. Lippincott.

McFarlane, J., Greenberg, L., Weltge, A., & Watson, M. (1995). Identification of abuse in emergency departments: Effectiveness of a two question screening tool. *Journal of Emergency Nursing, 21* (5), 391–394.

McGregor, N., & Barnet, V. (1998). Personal communication.

Miller, J. (1995). Caring for Cambodian refugees in the emergency department. *Journal of Emergency Nursing, 21* (6), 498–501.

Miller, L. (1996). *Trauma: ED to ICU*. Conference with handouts, Syracuse, NY.

Murphy, K. (1997). *Pediatric triage guidelines*. St. Louis: Mosby-Year Book.

National Institute on Alcohol Abuse and Alcoholism (1997). *Alcohol alert: Alcohol-related impairment*. No. 38. Rockville, MD: U.S. Department of Health and Human Services.

National Institute on Alcohol Abuse and Alcoholism (1994). *Alcohol alert: Alcohol-related impairment*. No. 25 PH 351. Rockville, MD: U.S. Department of Health and Human Services.

Nettina, S. (1997). *Lippincott's pocket manual of nursing practice*. Philadelphia: Lippincott-Raven.

Newark/Wayne Community Hospital (1992). *Emergency department triage manual*. Newark, NY: Author.

New York State Department of Health (1994). *Sexually transmitted disease: Treatment guidelines 1994*. Albany, NY: Author.

New York State official compilation of codes, rules, and regulations (1994). Albany, NY: Lenz and Riecker.

Nugent, K., et al (1988). A model for providing health maintenance and promotion to children from low-income, ethnically diverse backgrounds. *Journal of Pediatric Healthcare, 2* (4), 175–180.

Nursing 82 photobook: Working with orthopedic patients (1982). Springhouse, PA: Intermed Communication.

Nursing 84: Emergencies (1985). Springhouse, PA: Springhouse.

Nursing Update (1975). Religion and patient care: Beliefs that can affect therapy. 6–9.

Orgue, M., et al (1983). *Ethnic nursing care: A multicultural approach*. St. Louis: C.V. Mosby.

Overfield, T. (1985). *Biologic variation in health and illness: Race, age, and sex differences*. Menlo Park, CA: Addison-Wesley.

Pediatric advanced life support (1994). Dallas: American Heart Association.

Pfeiffer, W. (1994). *Technical writing: A practical approach*. New York: Macmillan.

Rayan, G., & Flourney, A. (1995). Hand infections. *Contemporary Orthopaedics, 20* (1), 41–53.

Remington-Klein, A., Lee, G., Manton, A., & Gren-Parker, J. (1994). *Emergency nursing core curriculum*, (4th ed.). Philadelphia: W.B. Saunders.

Roberts, C. (1997). Focus on thrombolytic therapy for acute ischemic stroke. *Heartbeat: A Cardiac Nursing Newsletter, 7* (2), 1–11.

Roper, M. (1996). Back to basics: Assessing orthostatic vital signs. *American Journal of Nursing, 96* (8), 43–46.

Ruiz-Contreras, A. (1995). Thoughts on labels from a Chicano emergency nurse. *Journal of Emergency Nursing, 21* (6), 515–516.

St. Joseph's Hospital (1993). *Emergency department triage manual*. Syracuse, NY: Author.

St. Mary's Hospital. (1994). *Emergency center triage protocols*. Rochester, NY: Author.

Santopietro, M. (1981). Indochina moves to Main Street: How to get through to a refugee patient. *RN Magazine,* January, 43–48.

Schmidt, R. (1988). *Exploring religion* (2nd ed.). Belmont, CA: Wadsworth.

Schmitt, B. (1980). *Pediatric telephone advice.* (1st ed.). Boston: Little, Brown.

Schmitt, B. (1994). *Pediatric telephone protocols.* Littleton, CO: Decision Press.

Selfridge, J. (1992). *Challenges in emergency nursing.* Philadelphia: W.B. Saunders.

Sheehy, S.B., & Barber, J.M. (1985). *Emergency nursing: Principles and practice.* St. Louis: C.V. Mosby.

Shives, L. (1990). *Basic concepts of psychiatric-mental health nursing* (2nd ed.). Philadelphia: J.B. Lippincott.

Shultz, S. (1982). How Southeast Asian refugees in California adapt to unfamiliar health care practices. *Health and Social Work,* 148–156.

Simoneau, J.K. (1985). Disaster aspects in emergency nursing. In *Emergency nursing: Principles and practice* (pp. 390–425). St. Louis: C.V. Mosby.

Sinclair, C. (1996). *Handbook of obstetrical emergencies.* Philadelphia: W.B. Saunders.

Smith-Suddarth, D. (1991). *The Lippincot manual of nursing practice* (5th ed.). Philadelphia: J.B. Lippincott.

Speedy Spanish for medical personnel (1980). Santa Barbara, CA: Baja Books.

Stern, P. (1990). Selected acute infections. *American Academy of Orthopedic Surgery: Instructional Course Lectures,* vol. 39, ch. 67.

Tardiff, K. (1989). *Assessment and management of violent patients.* Washington, DC: American Psychiatric Press.

Trauma nurse core curriculum (1991). Chicago, IL: Emergency Nurses Association.

U.S. Department of Health & Human Services (1990). *Sexually transmitted diseases summary.* Atlanta, GA: Public Health Service, Centers for Disease Control.

Understanding of child abuse and neglect needed (1993). National Research Council.

Varcarolis, E. (1998). *Foundations of psychiatric mental health nursing* (3rd ed.). Philadelphia: W.B. Saunders.

Varcarolis, E. (1994). *Foundations of psychiatric mental health nursing* (2nd ed.). Philadelphia: W.B. Saunders.

Walleck, C. (1994). Emergency nursing across the life span: Neurologic emergencies. *ENA Clinical Monograph Series, 1* (3).

Wiggins, M., et al. (1994). The management of dog bites and dog bites to the hand. *Orthopedics, 17* (7), 671–623.

Wolbert-Burgess, A. (1997). *Psychiatric nursing: Promoting mental health.* Stamford, CT: Appleton & Lange.

Wordsworth dictionary of beliefs and religions (1995). Ware, Hertfordshire: Wordsworth Editions.

Yamada, T. (1991). *Textbook of gastroenterology* (vol. 1, 2.) Philadelphia: J.B. Lippincott.

Index